Nursing

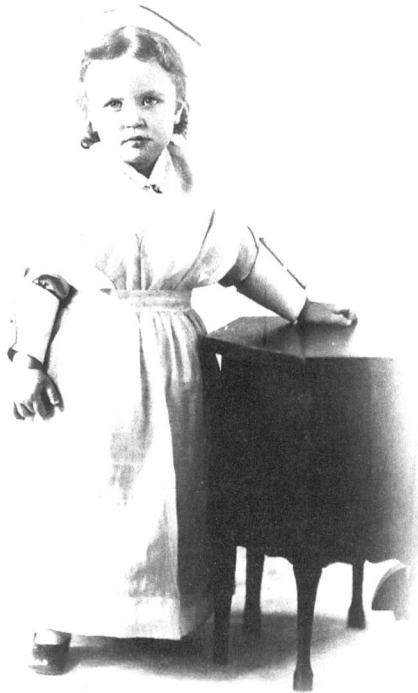

The Little Handbook
Of
Basic Essentials

How to be a Truly Great Nurse
~simply~ by
Providing Excellent Patient Care
∞ Lessons on Blending Art with Science at the Bedside ∞

Kathleen Jimenez RN

Nursing 101

The Little Handbook of Basic Essentials

How to be a Truly Great Nurse
~simply~ by
Providing Excellent Patient Care
∞ Lessons on Blending Art with Science at the Bedside ∞

The Author/Publisher has prepared this book to the best of her abilities and has intended to provide accurate and authoritative information with regard to the subject matter contained herein. However, she makes no representation as to the applicability or completeness of this book. Information and recommendations given are based on personal professional knowledge and experience only. No references whatsoever have been utilized in the writing of this book, other than the quotations by Florence Nightingale appearing throughout the text, simply as points of interest. As such, there are no citations to that end, other than the references to her work.

It is sold with the understanding that the Author/Publisher is not engaged in rendering legal, accounting, and/or other professional/clinical/ethical advice. If legal advice or other expert assistance is required, the reader should seek professional services to meet that need.

The Author/Publisher disclaims any warranties (express or implied), merchantability, or appropriateness for a specific purpose. This book contains material protected under International and Federal Copyright Laws.

The names and identifying details of any real persons have been eliminated to protect their privacy.

Dedication

This book is dedicated to my children—for enduring more of me than they should, and for all the joy they bring to my life amidst an endless supply of insanity.

Acknowledgments

My parents for creating an environment of self-actualization. My grandmother, Maggie, for being my rock in the storm—the greatest storyteller of all time with the best sense of humor on the planet...salt of the earth, strong beyond belief. Judy Johnson for sharing the wonder of "Making an Occupied Bed" with an awestruck 6 year old girl. I am pretty clear that **may** have been the reason I chose Nursing. Well, **that** and actor Chad Everett (Dr. Joe Gannon on "Medical Center")!

Cheryl, Judy, Ma and Pa—my second family.

Michael for allowing me to share the most **amazing** End of Life experience with his dad, Earl—and Rose, for choosing to have me at her side on the journey.

George Mason University for my degree and the opportunity to begin this journey as a Nurse Extern prior to graduation. Local Nursing was in a transient surplus at that time, and many of my classmates were unable to find jobs as New Grads. I was both grateful and humbled to just slide into mine on the very same floor where I had worked for 7 months.

Dorothy, Bonnie, Pat, Rita, Vicki, Julie, Gail, Gloria, Virginia, and Sue from T7W—1982-1985. A few of the Urology Boys (my favorites): Dr. Mike Manyak for calling me tenacious—the greatest compliment of my career; Dr. Gary Fialk for teaching me to grab it like a stick shift; Dr. Dan Laurent for his endless supply of funny stories and for always being such a gentleman. Dr. Patrick Carroll for his honesty in confronting a poor prognosis when others offered merely false hopes, citing **this** study or **that** statistic; for his insight regarding the effect of sugar consumption on promoting the growth of certain Cancers—way ahead of his time; also for throwing all straws in the trash on his post-op patients—**and**, not to forget, his delightful Irish Brogue. Likewise, Dr. Myron Berger for his disdain of Styrofoam cups.

Dr. Hector Ducci for genuinely appreciating that a very young 22 year old Nurse had an alcohol wipe in her pocket at just the right moment—and for those amazing good looks. Dr. William Byrne for his perpetually missing glasses which were usually on top of his head, and for acknowledging when my dear father-in-law died. Dr. Thomas Fulcher for totally shocking us all by kneeling up on the bed in his suit (no less) to pull up a patient requiring a 4-person lift.

Margie for nearly 3 decades of friendship and cheerleading. I love you. Thank you.
Cynthia and Jim for friendship and being my best editors and critics.
Tom and Nancy for being who you are...The Best.

Donna (aka the Grimster) for laughter and happy memories of exploding syringes, dripping Meds, hissing thermostats, afternoon tea-time, and countless other stuff—too much to mention. Now, where did I leave those Ray-bans! Mary for sharing the making of her baby quilt while working nights and for turning ICU bathtime into so much fun during *Friday Night* (Music) *Videos*. Shirley for being Shirley. Prince has no idea what he missed. Beth for being a friend at a really crummy time and my best pal for haunting Old Town.

Dr. Dean Glassman for making us coffee every morning at o'dark-thirty when we had all just about lost it while trying to stay awake in ICU4, **and** for not being afraid to read the instructions for inserting a Sengstaken-Blakemore Tube at the patient's bedside, just as we were about to do it. Dr. Frank Fusco for being an icon in all ways. Chairman of the Board, baby! Dr. George Bazaco for the best Baklava on the planet every Christmas (Thank You, Mother Bazaco!). Dr. Robin Goldenberg for his intellect, interest, and enthusiasm. I will forever remember the sight of you driving the Volvo to work one fine Spring morning—windows down, shades on, "Glory Days" blasting on your radio. Dr. Allan Morrison for his red dress dream. Dr. Donald Poretz who first gave life to the concept of "sweet-smelling sweat". Dr. Ernesto Castro for being such a charmer!

Dr. Paulo Franco for always leaving a trail of Giorgio for Men wafting through the halls. Dr. John Moynihan for knowing me as long as he has (you were Chief/I was a New Grad) and for being a kind and gentle Surgeon with steady hands (my gall bladder thanked you too!). Dr. Dan (the Man) Turgeon for being yet another great Resident, and later a great Attending. Dr. Mike Potter for identifying the somewhat unusual drainage from an abscess as "ectoplasm" at just the right moment—great comedic timing! Dr. Ed LeFrak and Dr. Alan Speir for letters of appreciation, and Dr. Speir (in particular) for his sincere and well-timed apology.

Pearl for giving me purpose, and Carl for bringing me joy and faith. Gigi for introducing me to Gold Cup-crashing and for bringing a steady stream of laughter to some rough days and nights in IMC. Joanne for some of the most unbelievable stories, like the horse and carriage ride on her honeymoon.

Brenda for being such a huge support, and Leighann for being herself. Lynn for being who she was—broom and all—she made me stronger. Jan for both her wisdom and her relentless focus on health and staying fit (not that I have always followed her example!). FFX Anesthesiologists for providing such a collaborative work environment and for great Christmas Parties (until they stopped).

Mary Jane Mastorovich for her brutal frankness. I will always remember, "If you don't like it, you can leave!" All the Nursing Supervisors, '82-'96. Sue Mosedale, most of all!

Dr. Glenna Andersen for delivering my boys—the best!

All my patients and their families from Home Care and Hospice. Totally unforgettable! Especially, Cmdr Tom C— forever soaring in the skies. Mr. D for coffee, pastry, and fresh figs plucked from his tree.

Lizzie...the best window washer a girl could ever have—a **truly** Great Nurse! And, did I tell you..."You're looking very very beautiful tonight!"

Joanne for being my other (Gold) half at IHH.

Linda, Becky, David, Madeline, Jeff, and any others who helped me keep my sanity at "Mecca"...Not! And to those who resisted change, you DEFINITELY made me stronger. Dr. Tom Daniel, Dr. Ivan Crosby, Dr. David Jones, and Dr. Irving Kron—the Virginia Boys—for 2 years that taught me a great deal about personal fortitude.

Nancy and Gayla for giving me the chance to come back to the best work on the planet. Dr. Tom Sullivan for genuine collaboration and consistent respect for my clinical judgment.

Luisa for being there through thick and thin...you are beautiful in all ways, and always!

Leila for giving me the chance to be a viper of an expert witness—what great fun!

The Oaks for giving me the chance to prove my theories. Judy and Marie for being there....I never would have made it those 18 months without you. Alex, Ann, Beth, Blessy, Carissa, Caroline, Cathie, Diane, Katrina, Kristin, Mary, Peggy, Renee, Stephanie, Vanessa and all the other Oaks friends. Dr. Mark Franke and Dr. Munish Goyal for your commitment to Evidence-based Medicine and Best Practice (despite forces to the contrary), for always taking your time with patients AND with Nurses—also, for your continued friendship.

My stones and my stent which gave me the opportunity to be at home and find my dream job.

Kelly and Meg for believing in me. Marianna, Eileen, and Barbara for your commitment and dedication to the profession.

R for showing me I CAN do it all on my own, and many others for revalidating that lesson.

And, most of all...Jeanne Maguire for giving me the opportunity to experience that which led to the writing of this book...my icon and my hero!

Table of Contents

Caveats: the Author has taken certain liberties with regard to traditional literary style, such as the capitalization of words specific to Nursing and/or healthcare for the purpose of highlighting their distinction. Likewise, she has selected certain gender designations to simplify her writing such as the consistent reference to the Nurse and Secretary as "she", the Physician or Doctor as "he", etc. This is in no way a sexist commentary; rather, it represents what was most typical at the time the Author began her career some 30+ years ago. Its purpose is nothing more than to ease not **only** the process of writing, but of reading, as well. Your understanding is appreciated in this matter. Please note also, Nursing is a language unto itself. Use this text as a primer to learn its nuances, whether you are a Student Nurse, a Nurse already in practice, some other type of healthcare administrator or provider, and/or even a patient or family member. Whatever your frame of reference, Nursing 101 provides a precise, time-tested, and easy-to-understand formula for the provision of excellent care. Many texts talk around and about the Art of Nursing, but this one jumps right into the deep end, and actually tells you how to swim to the other side, and **survive**! In fact, some non-Nurses have even high-jacked our own concepts only to then turn around and "teach" them to us disguised as the newest flavor of "sliced bread"—no thanks, not so much. We have GOT this, folks! Always have.

Prologue

So you **want** to be a Nurse. Or perhaps you **are** a Nurse, but no longer feel satisfied in your career. In either case, you must ask yourself the first essential question—"Do I *truly want* to be a Nurse?" If your answer is yes, then ask the second essential question—"Do I *truly know* what it is to be a Nurse?" The bottom line is—to be a truly *Great Nurse* **and** to feel fulfilled—you must answer these questions with a clear understanding of the commitment you are about to make—or may have made already.

For those of us with many years of experience, there are no illusions. Nursing is **Hard Work**. It always has been; it always will be. If you are not **prepared** for hard work, you are likely making the wrong choice. No amount of medical breakthroughs, technological advances, or streamlined systems will ever change the undeniable reality of Nursing. In **any** setting, Nursing is physically, mentally, and emotionally challenging. At times, it **may** even test your spirit.

You can be a *Hospital Nurse* with the most ideal staffing and still have a rough day. You can work in *Home Care* and face traffic jams, mountains of *Documentation*, and visits that run longer than planned—turning your eight hour day into twelve. You can work in a Doctor's Office or a Clinic with a phone and an appointment schedule that never end. You can work in a *Hospice* setting and give everything you have, yet still not be able to relieve someone's pain—nor ease their fear of death.

If you want to be a Nurse, there is no "safe" place. There is nowhere to hide out, pass the time, make a few calls, take a long lunch, blow out early on a Friday, or cruise in late on a Monday. Nursing does not tolerate an absence of commitment. It is a calling—not a career choice of default or second best. For most of us, second best will never be good enough. Your ultimate dissatisfaction will come through loud and clear to your patients. Shame on you and pity for them! You will have both missed an amazing opportunity to experience true and unforgettable humanity at its best.

Be absolutely certain Nursing is what you want—and then, *embrace* it! If you are not happy or at your best in one *Area of Clinical Practice*, try another! Find your place, but do not settle for professional misery. Do not make your patients suffer for your unwillingness to take charge of your personal satisfaction on the job. Nursing provides an opportunity few careers can offer—the ability to move around and about in so many diverse areas of practice, yet all under the umbrella of being a Nurse. There is no excuse to stay some*place*—or with some*thing*—if you are not fulfilled. Make another choice. It is **that** simple.

So assuming you have answered "yes" to the essential questions, you must first be able to stand the sight of blood and other bodily fluids. You must get through *Nursing School* and pass your *Boards*. You must choose an area of clinical practice and find yourself a job. Beyond **that**, there are some simple (though not always easy) *Steps* that you absolutely **must** follow. In the case of those who are already Nurses, you may have missed this final ingredient for success. Yet— whether just starting out, or even starting over—it can be done. The trick is to be clear and to commit—as much to the principle, as to the process.

The purpose of these Steps is to provide a set of sequenced fundamentals demonstrating clarity in thought and action through utilization of the *Nursing Process*, as a familiar roadmap for success. They represent the essentials of patient care, and should be the framework for *Nursing Practice* in any clinical setting. To *Assess*, Plan, Act, and Evaluate is a format with applications to all that we do in Nursing—not just care at the bedside. It is with that in mind that these Steps have been defined. They are by no means exhaustive. Any survey of a roomful of well-seasoned Nurses would undoubtedly reveal many more secrets and suggestions. **But**—these are the basics which provide a solid foundation for developing one's own style in both the *Art and Science* of being a Nurse.

These Steps are more specific to Hospital Nursing and carry a few critical assumptions. The absence of one or more of these assumptions may change the dynamics of your ability to follow certain of these Steps; but, follow them you must. They include, but are not limited to:

o   You work in a healthcare facility or system that you can support and which likewise supports you.
o   You have a boss who is fair, direct, knowledgeable, honest, *AND* in whom you trust.
o   You are absolutely clear about the area of Nursing in which you have chosen to practice.
o   You are able to come to work each day having checked all of your personal baggage at the door when you walk in.

Do not bring your troubles into the hospital, unless it is to talk over with a friend in private on a break with a cup of coffee. Under no circumstances should you ever burden your patients with your own issues—personal or professional. They are not there to be your confidant, your advisor, your sounding board, or your advocate. If you have made a clear and conscious decision to become a Nurse, it is incumbent upon you to put on a happy face when you walk through the door to work. No exceptions. No substitutes. No patient lying ill in a hospital bed wants to see sad or angry faces, nor hear the gripes and complaints of the people responsible for his or her care.

Yours is to care for, to nurture, to comfort, and to console. With all the technology, Documentation, *Coordination of Care*, and everything else that pulls you away from your patients—to be a truly Great Nurse, you must never forget that which is the essence of Nursing. To be able to sit at someone's bedside, take their hand, and ask them their story is the unique privilege of Nursing. It is not **just** about *Medications* and *Vital Signs* and *Charting*. It is about changing the day—and many times the life—of another human being with a single interaction. THAT is Nursing, my friends!

"I use the word nursing for want of a better. It has been limited to signify little more than the administration of medicines and the application of poultices. It ought to signify the proper use of fresh air, light, warmth, cleanliness, quiet, and the proper selection and administration of diet — all at the least expense of vital power to the patient."

Florence Nightingale
Notes on Nursing, 1859

The Twelve Steps for Being a Great Nurse

Introduction

The roots of these so-called "Steps" are nothing more than common sense mixed with care, compassion, and coordination. They do not represent Rocket Science. Many organizations have adapted elements of these Steps, labeling them with catchy phrases and clever acronyms. They typically use them as part of a program of *Service Excellence* to improve *Patient Satisfaction Scores*. Likewise, they hope to enhance their reputations—and ultimately, their bottom lines—a necessary reality in today's world of healthcare. *AND*, that is all well and good if patients truly benefit from those efforts; however, their purpose is something deeper and far more significant than notoriety or financial gain as hopeful by-products of *Clinical Excellence*.

What is most critical about these Steps is the enhancement of human caring through astute attention to detail and a defined systematic process—*ALONG WITH* the elements of kindness, respect, and communication. None of this is new or different. These concepts have been the bedrock of Nursing Practice since its inception. Yet for a variety of reasons, they have slipped away—weakening the stability of our profession. It is time to refocus our philosophy, our practice, our teaching, ***and*** our commitment on such fundamentals.

These Steps apply no matter where you work in the hospital setting, from one in-patient unit to another. Yet they can also be adapted to an out-patient setting such as the *Emergency Department* or the *Post-Anesthesia Care Unit (Recovery Room)*. You will even find them helpful in a community setting such as Home Care or Hospice. Essentially—no matter where you practice in Nursing, you **must** develop a routine that works. The specific details of how you perform your duties may be dictated by the *Model* through which patient care is delivered in your particular area of practice—however, it is surprisingly easy to be successful from one to the next with nothing more than a commitment to such basic essentials.

So whatever the terminology—and whatever the patient population—the message is the same. It is through ***these*** Steps that Nursing is at its best. It is by using ***this*** process that patients are given the most excellent care they can receive. They follow the logical progression of a day in the life of a Nurse and her patients on any given shift. The old adage to keep it simple is based on fact and effective results. That is about as tough as it gets. **Just do it!**

Step One
Get to work early and on time.

Are you confused? Which is it? Early? Or on time? Well, if it is not one, it had best be the other! Essentially, this means getting to work no later than 0645 if your shift starts at 0700, or by 1845 if your shift starts at 1900—that is 7 a.m. and 7 p.m., for all you civilians. Ideally, you would do better to get there a half hour **before** your start time. You will then be able to put away your things, get a cup of coffee, and socialize for a few minutes. After that, you must quickly determine your assignment so you can pull together your "papers", your documentation, or whatever it is you need to begin your day or night. Not to mention, it is only fair to the shift that is leaving. After all, how would you feel if the oncoming shift strolled in late? Remember the *Golden Rule*? This is one of those times.

We all know the stress that arriving late can (or should) cause. Why get off to a bad start? It is inevitably a much better feeling to arrive ahead of time, take a moment to breathe, collect your thoughts, and start your shift with a sense of calm and control—rather than breathless fear and anxiety. If you have no sense of the inappropriateness of coming in late, do not bother reading on. Make another choice and do us all a favor. Save yourself and those around you the burden of your carefree attitude. There is no place for it in Nursing—especially in the hospital setting. Not to mention, there is likely a policy pertaining to when you **should** clock-in before the start of your shift. Find it, and know what it is.

While being a "free spirit" may work for you in some areas of Nursing, it must always be tempered by an utter sense of responsibility and duty that are most often extremely time-sensitive. There are few technical aspects of clinical practice at the bedside not driven by time. If you choose a career path with any degree of direct patient care, you will need to commit to watching the clock. A purely clinical tract in almost any setting is based on schedules and precisely timed interventions. In *Nursing Leadership*, it is also about time and routines and schedules—not only yours, but also those of your staff. As a *Nurse Educator*, you cannot stroll in to teach your class whenever the mood strikes. The sooner in your decision-making to become a Nurse that you determine the degree of your innate ability for timeliness—or its absence—the better off you will be.

Essentially—if you are not about attention to time and detail, Nursing is probably not the career for you. Better to know that early on, rather than later when you are miserable and cannot figure out why. In fact, you would be lucky to get through

Nursing School without a tremendous capacity for self-discipline and time management. **But**—be prepared! While you may not have to study as much, and might have fewer *Care Plans* to write, your need to watch the clock will not diminish once you graduate and complete your formal education.

In truth, you should learn something new every day you are a Nurse throughout your entire career—even if it is only a validation of what you already know or believe to be true. Never become complacent with your base of knowledge. On any given day, if all you learn is how to improve your time management by one small step, you will have grown and enhanced your practice—leading to greater satisfaction for both you and your patients.

"I never lose an opportunity of urging a practical beginning, however small, for it is wonderful how often in such matters the mustard-seed germinates and roots itself."

Florence Nightingale
Letter to a friend, quoted in The Life of Florence Nightingale Vol. II (1914) by Edward Tyas Cook

Step Two
Find a System that works and stick to it.

Wherever you work in Nursing—but especially in the hospital where there is so little within your control (in spite of your responsibility to control it all)—you need to find, develop, beg, borrow, or steal a *System* for setting up your day (or night) that works and allows you to roll with the punches that inevitably come. You need to be able to get your work done, ensure that your patients are cared for (and feel the same), yet still walk out the door by a reasonable time at the end of your shift. Be creative. Look to your peers. Find someone who gives excellent care and ask them how they organize their work. Try it. See if it works for you. If so, embrace it as your own or keep searching until you find the right fit. **But**—without exception—you **must** have a System.

Whether it is a form you create, a list you make, a chart, a schedule, whatever—you need to have a routine way of organizing your work, keeping track of information and tasks to be done, and a method for tending to your patients so that nothing is missed. Critical to a job well done—and a sense of both personal and professional satisfaction—is that you **and** your patients feel you have given your best. No matter how great your hospital's *Documentation System*—nor how useful your *Kardex* or Care Plan—the truly **Great** Nurses have a System and stick to it—no matter what.

Ideally, you should develop a routine for everything you do in Nursing that goes beyond just following your hospital's *Policies and Procedures*, such that it becomes ingrained in your mind and a natural part of your daily habits on the job. Once you become proficient as a Nurse, certain aspects of your practice should simply be second nature. The only way to achieve proficiency is to learn the steps for doing something right, and then to do it—over and over until it becomes rote. Once you are competent, you may be better able to see where a process could (or should) be changed to increase efficiency—or to achieve a better outcome.

Flexibility is also a key element in Nursing, but it must always be grounded by a strong foundation of having developed a routine, and then following it **every single day**. The easiest way to do this is by finding a role model and adapting their style to your own. Anywhere you go in Nursing, there will always be one (and hopefully more than one) truly **Great Nurse** who seems to have it all together. Latch on and see what she does. You really **can** learn a lot through someone else's experience. Later—when you have mastered the basics—you can develop your own style a bit more so that you will be ready when it is your turn to teach someone new. The time will come—believe it or not—when you will be viewed as the expert. Be confident; you **will** get there!

"The most important practical lesson than can be given to nurses is to teach them what to observe."

Florence Nightingale
Notes on Nursing, 1859

Step Three
Know what you are supposed to know.

Beyond the obvious of knowing what your assignment is, you need to listen attentively to *Report* and ask questions if it is verbal. If your Report is taped, seek out the off-going Nurse for clarification. (P. S. She had better still be there, tending to the patients while you listen to the tape.) The *Best Practice* is to give Report at the bedside, as you make *Walking Rounds* together—**before** you take over and she is out the door. There has probably never been a Report in the history of Nursing that was 100% complete. There is always something missing and you should be astute enough to recognize that and ask the questions that need to be asked.

In addition, make it a habit to look at your patients' *Charts* before you ever walk down the hall or pass a Medication. Even if you have 6 or 7 patients, it really only takes a few minutes to open a Chart, look at the last *Progress Note* and the *Doctor's Order Sheet*. Do they match? Was something that was referenced in the Progress Note followed through on as a plan in the Orders? If not, ask **why** not.

Did he (the Physician) say he was going to "Transfuse 2 Units of *PRBCs*", but only ordered a "*Type and Screen*"? Did he refer to "*Discharge Planning*" as being in progress, but never ordered a Social Work, Case Management, or Discharge Planning Consult? If it takes 15 or 20 minutes, it may save you an hour or two later on for something that would have been missed. You will start out your shift knowing what the Doctor's plan is, so that you can adjust yours accordingly.

Another advantage to checking your Charts immediately after Report is that if you find Orders not yet noted by the off-going shift, you may still have the opportunity to have her sign off and implement Orders that should have been already initiated—**assuming** she has not yet clocked out and left the building. Mind you, the *Best Practice* (again!) would be to go through your Charts with the Nurse giving you Report as you discuss each patient, prior to the Walking Rounds referenced earlier.

Why do someone else's work and have your patient suffer a further delay in treatment as well? Granted, in some hospitals, with the high volume of rounding Physicians, it is not always possible to gather all your Charts together at one time; **but**—if you can—*DO* it! Physicians will quickly learn the routine, and will seek you out to obtain the Chart. This can also facilitate an opportunity for face-to-face discussion about their particular patient, at just the right moment—namely, as you are giving Report to the on-coming Nurse. How great is that!

If you work in a system with *Computerized Physician Order Entry*, adapt this step to ensure that all Orders have been initiated, verified, or whatever the case may be in your particular Model of Care. However you get it done, the message is the same. Do not take on the responsibility of someone else's oversight or neglect. Make sure the off-going Nurse did all she **should** do, and if not, that she brought it to your attention—with an acceptable explanation for the delay. If *EVERYTHING* is in the computer—in terms of the patient's record—integrate that into this process as well.

Accountability is *HUGE* in Nursing. It is not about blame; but it is about providing the care that is ordered and needed in a timely manner. A rare missed order is *ONE* thing. A Nurse who **consistently** misses Orders and/or delays in some aspect of patient care is quite another. If you sense a pattern in one of your peers, address it with them directly, via the process known as *Peer Review*. If you do and it cannot be solved, you will need to seek support, but do not ignore the problem and do **not** put yourself in a position of liability for someone else's oversight (or neglect).

Hospital Nursing—in particular—is a 24/7 job, such that it is never *ALL* done. However, communication from one Nurse to the next about what is **left** to be done is absolutely critical for excellent patient care. One small omission can lead to countless negative outcomes for your patient. These may include the potential for pain and/or other suffering, an extended length of stay, as well as added costs for medical interventions that might not have been necessary. So much of this can be avoided with pristine attention to detail and thoughtful timely communication from one team member to the next. This applies to all members of the team, not just Nurses. You should expect the same standard of communication from everyone involved in the care of the patient—no matter what. If that is not happening, you must again seek support in facilitating those expectations across all departments.

What you **should** recognize is that the Nurse **is** (or should be) the hub of the wheel around whom all things turn—in terms of patient care. Clearly, the patient is the *true* center, but must rely on the Nurse to be his or her advocate. It is your job to coordinate every aspect of your patient's care on your shift, and to facilitate the plan for the oncoming shift. To spend 8 or 12 hours with a patient, and **not** know their *History*, *Current Condition*, or *Plan of Care* is to seriously miss the boat as a Nurse. All of this is yours to do, to know, to interpret, and to integrate. The list goes on and on. This may seem a tall order; if so, please refer back to the Prologue—Nursing is ***Hard Work***!

The Nurse **is** (and should be) the link between the patient and the care that surrounds the patient. A Great Nurse has it all under control with the knowledge and skill to make a patient's stay in the hospital a smooth ride. In fact, a patient who has received excellent care may just want to stay in the hospital longer than necessary. However, a not-so-good Nurse can leave a patient and their family feeling bewildered and wanting nothing more than to be discharged and get home to where they can care for themselves—or be cared for by family. That should ***never*** be the case in ***any*** setting in Nursing.

Just as it is your responsibility to provide excellent care, so too is it yours to know (not just assume) that your patient and family are satisfied with their care. The only way to do that is to ask. This should be done at least every day (if not every shift), and *CERTAINLY* prior to Discharge. It may feel awkward at first, but with practice, the process will quickly become second nature—"So, Mr. Jones, how are things going with your care? Are we exceeding your expectations?"

You may find that your hospital uses specific "trigger" words (related to patient satisfaction) which typically tie in to the post-discharge survey. Learn what they are and incorporate them into your "script" or basic routine. Role-play with a coworker if necessary, but you must develop some skill and grace with this process. Would you not want to know in real time that a patient had a concern with your care—rather than later, when it has become a formal Complaint or *Grievance* to which you must provide an official response?

Nursing is a tremendous responsibility. Most other members of the team come and go, spending only brief moments with the patient. The Nurse is often the only constant during the patient's stay. Yet sadly, the advent of alternate shifts and scheduling patterns has done much to eliminate that continuity, leading to the now-typically fragmented care in the hospital setting. Gone are the days when a patient had virtually the same Nurses on each shift for their entire admission. In fact, some hospitals rotate the assignment every 4 hours, creating dissatisfaction for the patient, as much as for the Nurse—not to mention the tremendous liability and potential for error or omission inherent in so many *Handoffs in Care*.

If you discover that fragmentation is the norm on your unit in the way assignments are made, be an advocate for looking at other possibilities. Never be timid about speaking up to suggest a better process or practice. This is *YOUR* job and *YOUR* workplace; *OWN* it! Be respectful and follow the *Chain of Command* in facilitating change, but do not be shy about promoting efficiency—and ultimately, excellence. This can be done in a variety of forums—staff meetings, a suggestion box, partnering with your direct supervisor, or better yet—through your hospital's model of *Shared Governance* (assuming they have one).

Be responsible and take accountability for constantly striving for the best possible work environment—in all matters. This may include the fundamentals of how patient care is organized, how assignments are made, etc. One simple suggestion can transform the workload—and ultimately the outcomes—on a massive scale. Never underestimate your personal power to effect necessary change. If your motives are driven by excellent patient care, you will never go wrong.

"I think one's feelings waste themselves in words; they ought all to be distilled into actions which bring results".

Florence Nightingale
Letter to a friend, quoted in The Life of Florence Nightingale (1913) by Edward Tyas Cook

Step Four
Take a tour and see what is happening.

Before you go running off in ten different directions doing what you **think** needs to be done, make *Rounds* on your patients and see what **really** needs to be done. This is a critical first step to starting your shift after you have taken Report and checked all of your Charts. Beyond the obvious benefit of knowing that all your patients are breathing and have a heartbeat, you may find that what you **thought** was needed is really **not** necessary, while something else may come as a pleasant (or sometimes unpleasant) surprise that requires your more immediate attention. Either way, it is better to know sooner rather than later.

After all, your priorities should be based on what your **patient** needs, **not** what you need. In the long run, it will make your job easier. An important point is that these Initial Rounds do not have to take a couple of hours or get you off track. You should knock on the door, announce your arrival, and then graciously enter the room while greeting your patient by name. This greeting should not be their first name, unless they have given you permission to do so—and never by "Hon" or "Sugar" (and not even "Dear")—the reason should be obvious! Tell them your name and introduce yourself as their Nurse for the coming shift. Then, take a detailed—though rapid—overview of the state of each patient and their environment.

o Do they need to be groomed or straightened in bed?
o Do they need ice or water or should it be taken away?
o Is the overbed table ready for the next meal?
o Is their phone within reach?
o Can they get to their call bell?
o Do the lights need to be off or on?
o Is the TV on the channel they want to watch or do they want it turned off?
o Is their *IV* running at the correct rate, and are the tubing and bag labeled?
o Are they in pain or discomfort?
o Is all equipment working as it should be?
o Is their bed in the proper position?
o Is the room looking like a disaster?
o Are they and/or their family feeling as though their needs are being met and their questions answered?
o Tell your patient and/or their family that you are just coming on duty and making your Initial Rounds.

o Tell them what the plan is as you know it to be for the day or night.
o Briefly review any instructions they need to know, like being *NPO* or calling for help before getting out of bed.

Obviously, if there is something that you or the patient identify as an immediate or critical need, *DO* stop and take the time to address it. Get it off your list—and theirs. You will both feel better for it. But for the most part, you are making a mental note—and written, if that prevents you from forgetting—of what the priorities are for *ALL* of your patients once you are ready to get down to business with each individual. Also, it allows you to determine what tasks can be delegated to a *Nursing Assistant* or *Tech*—if you are lucky enough to have one.

Likewise, if you *DO* have an Assistant or Tech, listen to report together, and make these Initial Rounds together as well. That simple action immediately establishes the perception of coordinated Teamwork in the eyes of the patient and/or family. Plus, it fosters the required *Delegation* that must occur between the Nurse and any assistive personnel involved in providing patient care. Finally, it also affords you a ready partner for tending to any urgent issues that cannot be handled by just one person as you go room to room.

In almost any hospital setting—including the *ICU*—there is no need to rush in and immediately perform a lengthy head to toe assessment on each one of your patients without first assessing the overall state of your entire assignment. They have been (or should have been) cared for up until the minute you arrived—and actually, until you have accepted responsibility for their care from the off-going shift after hearing Report. It is always better to check on **all** your patients in a brief rounding format so that you have an idea of the overall picture. Check the state of the forest before you analyze one tree, as you may have a smoldering fire somewhere, ready to ignite.

Again, this should **not** be a tedious process. With practice, you should be able to get through it in 30 to 40 minutes, depending on the size and acuity of your assignment—but you need to be moving and observing and taking in everything all at once. When done right, you should appear graceful and in control. You should exude confidence and organization, not chaos and crisis management. Remember, the tone for your entire shift is set with the patient and/or family during these initial interactions. Make a good first impression!

Likewise, **demonstrate** to the patient and family that you and your coworkers are functioning like a well-oiled machine, in terms of Teamwork. Two (and even three) people sweeping into a room, working in unison to tidy up both the patient and his/her environment, attending to any immediate needs, and performing a brief but thorough assessment of any issues, concerns, or requests will send a HUGE message of competence, coordination, and caring. Again, this technique can (and **will**) work in virtually *ANY* area of clinical practice from an inpatient unit to the Emergency Department. Develop a name for this portion of the Rounding process, such as "Swarming" or "Buzzing". Use it as a code word for springing into action after hearing report. These simple techniques form the basis for motivation and camaraderie. Never underestimate their power—or the positive impression they will make on your patient and their family.

"The only English patients I have ever known refuse tea, have been typhus cases; and the first sign of their getting better was their craving again for tea."

Florence Nightingale
Notes on Nursing, 1859

Step Five
Be Prepared.

Taken in concert with Step Four, Being Prepared is a broad category and has many meanings depending on the setting in which you work, but requires essentially the same process. After hearing Report and checking your Charts, you should have a pretty good idea of what you will be doing for the day or night. You must now be certain you have what you need to do it.

- o Will you be doing wound care? Do you have all your supplies?
- o Do you have a patient with an *NG Tube*? If so, do you have a *Toomey Syringe*, *Normal Saline*, and a *Graduate* at the bedside? Are they labeled? Do you have a suction setup and is it working?
- o Do you have a patient with a *Feeding Tube*? Do you have enough of the formula that is ordered?
- o Do you have enough gowns, gloves, and masks for a patient in *Isolation*?
- o Does your patient have a bedpan and a *Washbasin* with toiletries in the bathroom? Are they labeled?
- o Check your Medications. Do you have the next IV *Infusion* in the refrigerator and/or all of your scheduled antibiotics or IV *Additives*?
- o Do you have the required bedside emergency equipment? Most often dictated by your area of clinical practice and/or patient condition. This may include such items as a Bag Valve Mask/Ambu Bag (basically, used to provide breaths during CPR or post-anesthesia when a patient is waking up but still needs support); suction and the associated supplies; wire cutters for a patient whose jaw is wired shut, and could need to be "unwired" quickly; an obturator, used for a patient with a tracheostomy (device through their neck into the trachea that allows them to breathe), in case the "trach" comes out accidentally—kind of a place holder if you will, until a new trach can be inserted—the backup trach should also be at the bedside.

The time you take to do this at the start of your shift will save you hours of phone calls and aggravation later on, and/or could save your patient's life. All of these items should be checked as you make your Initial Rounds—both **in** your patient rooms **and** at the Nurses Station, or in the Medication Room. Again, having a "System" will make this process easier. This is what lays the foundation for *Critical Thinking*. You should be going through a mental checklist as you enter each patient's room, just like a pilot preparing for takeoff. If you dart around the room without any appearance of organization or planning, that is exactly how you will look to your patient and/or their family. It will not instill any sense of confidence or coordination and will leave them feeling insecure and uncertain.

Furthermore, if you fail to take it all in when you first enter the room—focusing on only one or two aspects of their care—you will definitely miss out on things that will add time and frustration to your work. This will undoubtedly leave both you and your patient feeling that the day or night could have gone better than it did. You will be behind from the start of your shift and will most likely spend the rest of your time trying to catch up. Compound that with arriving late—in case you missed out on Step One—and you have the beginnings of a really rough shift. The solution is easy; the hard part is making the commitment with dedication and consistency.

Again, if you are making these Initial Rounds with your Assistant or Tech as recommended in Step Four, this is the perfect opportunity to create a plan related to those items to be delegated. Provide them with a list of those things with which they can help in relation to what was found on your Initial Rounds.

- Are there supplies missing from the room that they can gather?
- Do you need additional linen to perform a necessary but unexpected cleanup and bed change?
- If you do not have a formalized process for "passing ice and water" on your unit, could they do that once the two of you have finished rounding together on all of your patients?
- If one of your patients simply "does not look right", do you need an immediate set of Vital Signs as one component of a *Reassessment* in response to a potential change in condition?

The possibilities are endless as to what might be needed based on your Initial Assessment of the patient and/or family and their immediate needs. One caveat to this process is the *Staffing Plan* on your unit and the associated Model by which patient care is organized and delivered. More often than not, one Assistant or Tech may be shared between multiple Nurses. If such is the case, you may have to **modify** this process, as Initial Rounds **should** be made simultaneously by all Nurses on any given shift.

In that instance, your Assistant or Tech might need to make their own rounds and may not be able to accompany any one particular Nurse. If so, you will need to find a time and establish a process by which you regroup as soon as possible to review the patient assignment and those tasks to be delegated. Likewise, you will need to reconvene throughout the shift to monitor progress and results for **all** tasks completed and/or what may exist as an impediment to completing any one particular item. **Remember**, the Nurse is ultimately responsible for *ALL* care, delegated or not. You must close the loop by monitoring the Assistant's or Tech's work—to its completion. Period!

In the "olden" days of Nursing, Team Nursing was most often the norm—especially, when "wards" were larger and/or without doors. Even as late as the 1970's-80's, one "side" or "zone" or "hall" might be cared for by a pair or "Team" of Nurses—with or without an Assistant or Tech. Frequently, these Nurses made Initial Rounds together and utilized that time to attend to the immediate needs of the patients *TOGETHER*—to pass ice or water, and possibly even to take an initial set of Vital Signs. Such an approach made it possible for everyone to have "laid eyes" on the patients, so that in the case of an unexpected event, all could "pitch in" with a greater awareness of each individual patient. Even if your Model of Care has two Nurses partnered with one Assistant or Tech, make Rounds together as a Team. Imagine what could be accomplished for the benefit of the patient if three caregivers were to "Swarm" a room together. It **is** possible, and it can (and does) work!

Essentially, the key to any process in Nursing is to maximize efficiency while optimizing outcomes. Such should be the premise of any structure or hierarchy, anywhere you work. Be a visionary in your own right, and advocate for change when needed. Your patients always come first; everything else should be designed to meet their needs. Period! Yet so often, that is not the case, in terms of how things are organized, within the four walls of a hospital. Do not be discouraged. Take appropriate action.

Processes typically move in cycles within Nursing—often influenced by issues and constraints within healthcare in general. However, there is a **fundamental** body of knowledge surrounding Basic Nursing Care that is timeless. These elements should never be overlooked and/or excluded by Nursing Leadership and/or Hospital Administration when considering a new framework or Model of Care. Any failure to do so will undoubtedly result in poor compliance, marginal results, and low morale. Ultimately, most Nurses know the rules of safe and effective practice. It is the obligation of those in charge to ensure an environment which facilitates their success in applying those rules, rather than urging them to be abandoned for the sake of just getting through a 12 hour shift.

Essentially, if Nurses feel compelled to ignore what they know is best for the patient, it is typically the system itself that is broken. It is highly unlikely you will find a Nurse whose actual goal it is to provide poor care and/or leave her patients feeling dissatisfied! Inevitably, if that is occurring, there are only a few possible causes. Either the Nurse failed to correctly answer the fundamental questions of the Prologue (Do you truly want to be a Nurse? Do you truly know what it is to be a Nurse?). *And/or*, she was poorly trained in the first place. *And/or*, she is working in a hospital system run amuck. That is about as complex as it gets. While the latter is a huge issue to tackle, it can be done. However, it will require the single voice of Nurses to light the way.

"How very little can be done under the spirit of fear."

Florence Nightingale
Notes on Nursing, 1859

Step Six
Take a moment and regroup before you really get going, and at regular intervals throughout your shift.

Once you have made your Initial Rounds—assuming you did not find a crisis that altered the first hour or two of your shift—you should take a moment and rethink your plan. Inherent in this step is that you have a plan. If you do *NOT* have a plan, you should. You have heard Report, asked the questions, checked your Charts, **and** checked your patients. You should now have a better sense of what your priorities are—or need to be. Make the necessary adjustments to your thinking—*AND* to your System, especially if it is written. Be clear as to *WHO* or *WHAT* is first, second, and third on your list. Another point—at this particular juncture—is to take a minute and ask your peers how they are doing. Are they *OK*? Do they need any help? It is all about camaraderie and teamwork. When you need help, it will be more readily given if you have taken the time to help someone else when they have needed it. That old Golden Rule once again!

Again, this may be a perfect opportunity related to the process of Delegation described in Step Five. Gather your Assistant(s) or Tech(s) and strategize your plan. Include your fellow Nurses on the Team, especially if you share assistive personnel. Such a scenario demands that all Nurses on a shift collaborate to prioritize the care of **all** patients if there is only one Assistant or Tech, *OR* if each one is shared by multiple Nurses. Delegation requires that the Nurse prioritize the care to be given, delegated or not. As such, in the case of shared Assistants or Techs, the *RNs* on a shift **must plan and coordinate** to create a reasonable workload, **especially** when there are multiple critical needs. Do not place the Assistant or Tech in the position of feeling the need to decline a request due to being overwhelmed. This could easily be construed as *Insubordination*, when (in fact) it is nothing more than poor planning on the part of the Nurse (or Nurses).

Certainly, any Model of Care should have established routines delineating who does what, but this is *NOT* a substitute for the process of Delegation. The Best Practice would be a *Team Huddle* immediately after Initial Rounds. This provides an opportunity for all to validate the overall status of the unit (and *ALL* the patients) such that everyone is informed as to concerns, issues, and plans for the remainder of the shift.

Likewise, just as the responsibilities and priorities of the Nurse change throughout a shift in relation to the care of her patients, so too do the tasks of the Assistant or

Tech. They can easily become overwhelmed with multiple requests from more than one Nurse, and it is not theirs to determine the priority of what needs to be done. That remains the sole responsibility of the Registered Nurse.

In addition, there may be *LPNs* on your unit. This is another scenario where Delegation must be included in the process of making assignments and coordinating care. In most States, LPNs are limited in their practice related to some aspects of patient care. Be absolutely certain you know and understand the limits of their role, your own hospital's policy related to their utilization, and your professional responsibility in supervising their care.

Following the Team Huddle, when it comes to mastering Step Six, the value of "checking" cannot be overestimated. It is imperative to continuously evaluate your patients *AND* your progress with their care. Nothing can match that sinking feeling in the pit of your stomach at the end of a shift when you realize you have forgotten something critical. Likewise, perceiving yourself as so "busy" that you neglect to make **Hourly Rounds** on your patients may result in missing a subtle change in someone's condition that will alter the course of their care over the next 12 to 24 hours—or more.

As already referenced in Step Five, Step Six includes the need to check frequently with assistive personnel—again, **if** you have them. The foundation for teamwork and the key to quality patient care is communication. If you are working with an Assistant or Tech, do not forget to monitor their work. That is an essential component of Delegation. Once again, their duties should have been delegated by you, following your assessment of the patient and their needs. Likewise, you must assess your teammate and their ability to perform those tasks. Remember—you are ultimately responsible for all Nursing Care—delegated or not. Sound familiar? It **should**, by now. If **not**, you are clearly **not** paying attention!

To work with assistive personnel requires frequent checks as to what they have completed as well as their observations of the patient and/or the family. Your ability to value their input will optimize your professional relationship for the mutual benefit of the patient. You would be surprised how quickly patients and their families will perceive a lack of teamwork and communication among the caregivers on a unit. It sends the wrong message and will many times result in conflict and poor cooperation from the patient and/or family. Inevitably, you will spend more time trying to correct the perception than you would have spent by just taking the minute or two that is required to communicate and evaluate your work as a team.

Step Seven
Do not delay...just get started.

The fastest way to get off track is to get caught up in nonessentials once you have made your Initial Rounds. Perhaps you start socializing with someone you have not seen in a while; or you chat with a Doctor over something of interest, but not particularly pertinent. Once you have completed the first six Steps, it is time to begin and get on with your day or night. If you are following your System, you should be able to stay on track as you work through your shift. Make notes to yourself of items to be documented when you finally sit down to chart. Always note the time something happens so you can be accurate, and *ALWAYS* get the name of whom you are talking to for the inevitable follow-up as the shift goes on. The essence of time management in the hospital setting is to develop a routine and to stay on track. Again, this ties in to having a System and sticking to it.

It is imperative to develop a style in the organization of your work, the assessment of your patients, the documentation of your findings, and your process for responding to problems. If every day is like a blank slate, starting anew with a different approach, you will quickly burn out. More importantly, you will put your patients (and yourself) at risk for serious errors or omissions. The key is to stay focused. Do not dawdle or waste time when there are priorities to be met. Once you have assessed your patients, initiated your Medications or *Treatments*, **and** started your Charting, there is **always** time to interact with your peers and coworkers.

The key is to stay ahead of your schedule—**and** yourself. This is as simple as getting your "work" out of the way, early in the shift. The remainder of your time can be devoted to ongoing evaluations and course corrections with the Plan of Care as it evolves based on patient condition. Likewise, you will be busy with the implementation of timed Treatments, Medications, and new Orders. If you put off until the end of the shift what you could have (or should have) done at the start, you are setting yourself up for an hour or two of catch-up work long after everyone else has clocked out. Do not fall into this trap!

Surprisingly, a twelve hour shift can pass rather quickly. Coming out of the gait at the start of your shift without a plan and/or with a disorganized approach can only spell disaster. The nature of Nursing—especially in the Hospital —is that you just never know what may happen next. Being prepared, not wasting time, and staying on track are the essential ingredients for success. The key is consistency—**always**.

Step Eight
Check your Charts at regular intervals throughout your shift, and Note your Orders immediately.

Depending on your hospital's policy or practice, the *Unit Secretary* (*Health Unit Coordinator*) may **only** notify you of *STAT* orders—**OR,** not even that. It is always helpful if she **also** brings to your attention those Orders that are not STAT, but which are clearly time-sensitive, such as a Transfusion with a timed *H&H* to follow. If this is not done, you might make that suggestion to your Manager. It is just common sense to do so.

However—whether your Charts have flags, or if they are put in a certain location once the Orders have been entered by the Secretary—it is still up to you to check your patients' Charts and Orders on a regular basis. A routine *Chart Check* every 2 to 3 hours would be best. Formal Chart Checks should be completed at the end of each shift *AND* every 24 hours with a notation to that effect by the RN performing the check—and/or **always** with each Handoff in Care. Your hospital will (and should) undoubtedly have a policy addressing this fundamental *Standard of Care*.

Yet, no matter what your hospital's policy regarding timed Chart Checks, you should **always** verify that all Orders have been entered, requested, or—whatever system you use—that they have actually been initiated by the Secretary, in *REAL TIME*. Never assume that her initials or name on the page are a guarantee that the orders have been taken off correctly—or at all. Once you have signed your name, you are accepting responsibility for those Orders. You had better be sure they are done—and done right.

If there is a problem later on, it will not suffice to say that she signed off first. Do not fool yourself! **You** are the licensed personnel and it is incumbent upon you to supervise everyone, including the Secretary. If you find something is missing or incorrect, bring it to her attention with tact—but with clarity. Remember, the Unit Secretary is (or should be) your best friend. A good one can make your day. A not-so-good one can make your shift a virtual nightmare—not to mention what that will mean to your patients' care.

If you work in a system with Physician Order Entry, you can thank your lucky stars, but it is equally critical to review your computer printouts (or on-screen worklists) for accuracy and appropriateness. It is up to you to evaluate each Order in relation to the patient, and to question any Order that seems unclear or inconsistent with your knowledge of the patient and their needs. No matter the system, the responsibility rests with the Nurse for following Orders, *AND* for questioning those that you evaluate as being inappropriate.

An unfortunate by-product of Physician Order Entry has been a decrease in direct communication between Physician and Nurse regarding the Plan of Care—a fact more evident in certain hospital settings than in others. Not that a "paper" Chart was any guarantee of professional collaboration; however, our reliance on mechanized processes has clearly facilitated a less human approach. Be an advocate for face-to-face conversation regarding patient care. Do not allow this critical element of teamwork to take a backseat in the computer age. Active discussion is essential and your input is valuable and necessary for ensuring safe and effective patient care.

In addition—as you sign off or review Orders—make it a practice to read the Progress Note of the MD writing those Orders, as first described in Step Three. Beyond the possibility of finding an error or an omission, you will learn what his thinking is and (hopefully) any plan for the patient. Likewise, you will inevitably appear and sound much more knowledgeable—not only to the patient and their family, but to other Physicians who may be *Consulting*.

You can be informative and say, "Why yes, Dr. Smith was in to see the patient and he is considering…, or is planning to…" Of course, you must never reveal anything to the patient or family member that was not yet discussed by the Physician. Do not break that cardinal rule! That is not to say you cannot (or should not) advocate for the patient, and encourage the Physician to address some aspect of their care or condition—especially when he (the Physician) seems clearly reluctant to do so.

"No man, not even a doctor, ever gives any other definition of what a nurse should be than this — 'devoted and obedient.' This definition would do just as well for a porter. It might even do for a horse. It would not do for a policeman."

Florence Nightingale
Notes on Nursing, 1859

Step Nine
Document early, often, and accurately.

You absolutely must learn, embrace, and uphold the cliché that **if it is not documented, it was not done**. There is no room for discussion on this one. No matter what your hospital's system for documentation, you must develop your own personal method and discipline for Charting—and *STICK TO IT!* As you go about your shift providing care, make notes to yourself to be used later when you are ready to chart. If you have the ability to chart at the bedside with a computer in each patient's room, learn to do it.

If your hospital is computerized, and hopefully using a *Systems Format*, **be thorough**. *DO NOT* leave blanks and *DO* strive to be as detailed as possible. If you cannot include all you need to say in the space provided, add a *Narrative Note*. Be absolutely certain your computerized "checklist" charting matches any Narratives you may write, meaning do not just blindly check off "normal" for all assessment elements if there are actually negative findings to be documented. If you have an open Narrative paper Chart (i.e. a simple blank lined form), use the systems format here as well. It will keep you focused and ensure that you are less likely to miss something than if you just ramble on with no particular pattern or plan.

- o Always use correct terminology and only approved *Abbreviations*.
- o Always comment on your patient's Level of Consciousness, Orientation, and Communication.
- o Always describe their use of Glasses, Dentures, or Hearing Aids and the disposition of any of these items every time you care for the patient.
- o Always document their Vital Signs—as ordered—and for any change in condition.
- o Always assess for Pain and document your findings. No matter what your hospital's policy, a good rule of thumb is to assess at a minimum of every two hours, and certainly every time you interact with your patient—using a consistent *Scale*. Remember to *Reassess AND* Document their response to treatment after receiving pain medicine—and/or any other Medication used for symptom management.
- o Always listen to their Lungs and clearly document your findings. It is the only way you will ever develop any competency in doing so. The same applies to Heart Sounds.
- o Always check their extremities (arms and legs) for the presence/quality of pulses and the presence/severity of *Edema*.

o Always note their Diet and Appetite.

o Always, always, **always** validate their last *BM*—including the Amount and Character—and document the same, as well as the presence of Bowel Sounds and the condition of their Abdomen. In fact, that should be your **first** question whenever your patient complains of Nausea—when did you last move your Bowels? Likewise, if they complain of difficulty swallowing or a loss of appetite, check inside their mouth—they may have Thrush (yeast), especially among your Cancer patients, those with weakened immune systems, and post-antibiotic therapy.

o Always note their Urine Output, Character, and Color, as well as the *Mode of Urination*.

o Always note the condition of their skin (color, temperature, moisture, *Turgor*), along with the presence of any wounds—surgical, traumatic, or due to pressure (as in *Bedsores*).

o Always chart their Level of Activity and Mobility, along with the use of any *Assistive Devices*, and whether they belong to the patient or to the hospital. It will help you track when something is lost, if that should occur—and it often does; the same applies to those glasses, dentures, and hearing aids. In turn, your documentation (or lack thereof) may impact your hospital's obligation to reimburse the patient and/or family for items lost. To that end, be thorough. Many hospitals now issue a disclaimer to avoid financial liability for such personal items. However, if you document having taken possession of these things, the expectation will be to pay if lost.

o In addition, you will be documenting the presence of IVs, Drains, Tubes, etc. and the condition of each.

This is by no means an exhaustive list of basic assessment findings, but without these, you have nothing. Other things to document include:

o Any visits from family, friends, and Doctors

o Any trips off the unit to include where and why and the condition of the patient before and after transport, as well as how they were transported and by whom, i.e. via stretcher or wheelchair, as it is essentially NEVER appropriate to have a patient walk to their destination—especially at the time of Discharge; likewise, infants and children may be carried by the parent, but have the parent then ride in a wheelchair—the reason **should** be obvious! Many a permanent head injury was sustained by infants and children while "in the arms" of a parent who falls.

o Any time out of bed in a chair or ambulating (walking) and how it was tolerated as well as what level of assistance was required—complete assist, partial assist, contact guard, or independently—one person vs. two person, etc; with or without Oxygen (just be certain your actions correspond with Physician orders)

o Any interactions with the patient that reflect their mental or emotional state, or any other change in assessment

o Any and all safety measures based on any of a variety of assessment findings, events, or simply related to the reason the patient is in the hospital

While you must always document any incident or adverse event in concise factual terms, such as a *Fall* or a *Medication Error*, you must never refer to any sort of internal *Incident Report* in your notes. And, do not forget to document abnormal and/or critical lab findings or test results that have been communicated to you, along with what steps you have taken to notify the Physician, as well as any corresponding Orders you may receive—or a lack thereof. This is a regulatory standard—not optional.

One word of caution—in terms of documenting when Orders are **not** given, or for anything else that could be perceived as an error or omission—you must always document in a "neutral" manner. This means do not assign blame or in any way indicate neglect. Simply state, "MD informed. No Orders given." That is it! Never include words such as "refused" or "forgot" or anything else indicative of failure. Do not provide a roadmap for an Attorney, in the event of a negative outcome— especially when it may be completely unwarranted.

While you may (or should) have an instinct regarding actions to be taken in the case of an untoward event, and you **do** have an obligation to do everything within your *Scope of Practice* to ensure safe and appropriate care, so too should you never "point the finger" of blame at *ANYONE*—Physician, fellow Nurse, or any other member of the Team. If you are truly meeting with a "brick wall" when Orders are clearly indicated, seek the support of your Nursing Leadership.

Essentially, when it comes to documentation, if you follow your hospital's policies—as well as your own common sense—you should be fine. Almost always, more is better—as long as it is clear, factual, concise, consistent, and pertinent. With all handwritten documentation, never forget the critical importance of legibility. In the event of errors, omissions, or other incidents, your Notes may be the only tool you have to defend your actions when memory fails and/or there are conflicting accounts of what occurred.

Finally, in spite of the challenges of *Electronic Medical Record Systems*, never limit good documentation to a few disjointed Notes due to time or fatigue. If it means staying over after the end of your shift to accurately record the events that occurred, you **must** do so. The first time you are questioned regarding a patient's care will undoubtedly cure you of any reluctance to be thorough in this regard. Even when you had nothing to do with an incident, being deposed by an Attorney is something you will not (and should not) forget.

"If you find it helps you to note down such things on a bit of paper, in pencil, by all means do so. I think it more often lames than strengthens the memory and observation. But if you cannot get the habit of observation one way or other, you had better give up the being a nurse, for it is not your calling, however kind and anxious you may be."

Florence Nightingale
Notes on Nursing, 1859

Step Ten
Keep your patients informed at all times.

This goes along with the premise that you take the time to talk to your patients. Find out what they *do* know, what they *want* to know, and/or what they *need* to know. Share information with them in that regard, *if* it is appropriate to do so. If they are going for a test or procedure, explain it to them along with any instructions they will need to follow. Keep them informed as to when the test or procedure will be completed. *ALWAYS* tell them of any delays or cancellations. (P. S. If they have been NPO for a test or procedure and it has been cancelled or delayed, verify with the Doctor that they are able to eat and give them something as soon as possible—you will both feel better!)

Do not forget to identify yourself to the patient and clarify your role and responsibility in their care, along with that of any Assistant or Tech. This should have been done during your Walking Rounds at change of shift, and/or (again) during your Initial Rounds throughout your patient rooms. Validate that they know who their Physician is and why they are in the hospital. This is the foundation of your Nursing Assessment upon Admission, but it often bears reminders with some patients. This is especially true in teaching facilities and/or with multiple Consultants when there is an endless stream of care providers entering a patient's room throughout the course of a day. Be your patient's advocate in keeping the players straight.

Do not hesitate to invite yourself into the room—if the patient agrees—to serve as a "clinical" interpreter for what is being explained by the Doctor or medical team. As you should expect, patients are often overwhelmed when given information, and typically think of questions long after the Physician has gone—and frequently in the middle of the night, when sleeplessness leads to thoughts run wild. If you have been there to hear it first hand, you can have a significant impact on relieving their fears and calming their anxiety. You will be able to restate what was said by the Physician, and to further explain in layman's terms what was meant or intended. However, remember to **never** "break the news"—that is **not** yours to do.

One additional word of caution—when it comes to "interpreting" medical information, the act/process of obtaining *Informed Consent* might be perceived to fall into that category (erroneously, by the Physician). You must be clear—this is also *NEVER* yours to do. The Nurse must **never** obtain the patient's agreement (Consent) for a surgery or procedure as this requires a complete explanation of what is to be done, as well as the potential risks, benefits, and complications. If ever asked by a Physician to obtain Informed Consent, politely decline and provide him with the necessary form. Certainly, you can complete your portion, or fill in demographics, but—by regulations—this is his to do. Period!

It is especially important to close this loop of information at the time of Discharge. Do not let your patient leave without ensuring they understand what was done, what was found (if already stated by the Physician—it should have been, i.e. the Discharge *Diagnosis*), and what the plan is—as outlined by the MD in the *Discharge Instructions*. Again, **communication is the single most important tool in all aspects of effective patient care**.

Beyond those basics, there are many other categories of "information" pertaining to this Step.

o Upon admission, inform your patient and/or their family about the routines of your unit; how the shifts run (are they 8 hours or 12); explain who the caregivers are (a Nurse, an Assistant or Tech, etc.).

o Instruct them in the use of their phone, call bell, TV, and lights—along with any equipment related to their care which they must operate, e.g. the bed.

o Tell them how to order their meals, which will depend on their diet and the processes in your hospital (many hospitals have adopted a "Room Service" model by which patients may order their meals at any time of the day).

o Validate the reason for their admission, and *CLEARLY* explain when the Physician is most likely to see them. This is often the number one misperception—when they will be seen by the Doctor. Much of this depends on the severity of their illness, the unit on which they are a patient, and the model of Physician coverage in your particular hospital. In academic teaching hospitals, there is **never** a shortage of Residents and Interns; however, even **they** have their routines, and the initial visit by the Doctor is rarely immediate (except in critical care areas, such as the ICU—and, sometimes, not even there). Most non-academic hospitals employ (contractually) Doctors, known as Hospitalists, to see patients on behalf of private Physicians in the community. In either scenario, the bottom line is to do everything in your power to make this clear to the patient at the start of their stay, and to promptly communicate any delays (if possible) regarding the Physician's arrival on the unit.

o On a daily basis, and at the start of each shift, review the Plan of Care with your patient and/or family.

- o Ensure they understand the progress they are making along with other elements that may be impacting their ability to be Discharged.
- o In the case of delays (as already stated), be absolutely certain you give them a reasonable explanation as well as a realistic time frame for when a certain test or procedure **will** be completed. If there are changes, let them know immediately.
- o Before any care or bedside procedure, explain exactly what you will be doing—including how long it will take, what they may expect to see/feel/hear, anything to look for and/or report after it is completed, and *ALWAYS* allow them time for questions to validate their understanding. A classic method is to have the patient restate the information provided in their own words.
- o When administering Medications, open the package(s) and/or prepare the medicine at the bedside, explain its purpose(s) and any side effects the patient may expect and/or should report—as well as any safety precautions related to the anticipated/desired action of the Medication, such as using the call bell for assistance before getting out of bed following pain medicine that may cause sedation or dizziness, etc.

The essential lesson in Step Ten is to never assume that your patient (and/or family) knows or understands *ANYTHING*. However, do not be patronizing or condescending in your explanations. In fact, begin by asking them what they **do** know. This technique will allow you to tailor your explanations to their ability to understand—whether limited by age, education level, disability, or some other communication barrier—such as language, hearing, or sight. Seek guidance and utilize all available resources in this matter and document your actions to ensure understanding in the case of any defined barriers. When caring for pediatric patients, keep your explanation at a level that is age-appropriate, and include the parents (if available and/or willing) in your teaching.

The bottom line is to always make time to talk with your patients and/or their families. The impact of your efforts in this regard cannot be overestimated. You set the tone for your patient's entire stay with your initial interactions, and you reinforce that perception (good or bad) every time you enter their room and interact with them on a daily basis thereafter. Finally, be absolutely certain they end their stay with a good understanding of their condition, *AND* a great perception of you, your care, **and** your hospital or other healthcare setting. This can **only** be achieved by excellent communication. Master *THAT* and you are well on your way to success!

Step Eleven
Anticipate your patient's needs before they have to ask and stay ahead of yourself as much as possible.

The easiest way to please your patient and/or their family is to anticipate what they will need and to be on time with everything you do. This can be as simple as:

o Providing them the means to wash their face and hands prior to a meal or after using a bedpan or beside commode
o Clearing the way for their meal tray prior to its arrival
o Having the overbed table and their phone within easy reach at all times
o Anticipating their *PRN* pain medicine before the exact hour that it is due, so that if and when they do ask, you can say, "No problem, I can have that for you in just a minute!"
o Knowing they have just been given bad news by the Physician, and either want some privacy or a hand to hold

You will make their day—and yours. The more efficient and confident you appear, the greater their trust and cooperation. It really is that simple. Of course, there may always be one patient who cannot be satisfied no matter what you do. However, most patients will respond favorably to your sincere efforts to meet their needs by providing the care that is ordered in a timely and pleasant manner.

Furthermore, it is absolutely imperative that you put on a smile before you enter their room, no matter what. The fact that you were just yelled at by a Physician (not acceptable under any circumstance and can/should be dealt with), or that you have a patient who has soiled the bed 5 times in 2 hours, or that 3 admissions are coming at the same time, is not the problem or fault of any of your patients. None of them should be made to feel that it is. You can tell them nicely if you know you are going to be tied up for a while. But also—let them know that should they put on their call light, someone else **will** respond to their needs in your absence. It is also a wise idea to tell them when you are going "On Break" and who is covering for you. Someone should be! And—**always** ask your patient if there is anything you can do before you leave the room and tell them to call if they need you.

Associated with meeting the needs of your patient (especially when difficult to do) is the critical element of looking professional in **all** that you do—no matter what. Beyond the obvious of wearing a clean and proper uniform within the scope of your hospital's *Dress Code*, *AND* smiling whenever you enter your patient's room, you must also never allow your patient to become aware of the challenges and issues you may face related to getting the job done. The greatest *NEED* of your patient is to feel safe, secure, and well-cared for—your "face" and your behavior, as well as the attitude you convey with both, are what allows that to occur. You may have challenges with staffing or equipment, you may have a coworker who is not a team player, and the patient's Physician may not be responding to your calls or to his pager; *HOWEVER*, a truly **Great** Nurse *NEVER* allows the patient to perceive the stress these issues can create.

Another opportunity to look professional comes when "problem-solving" in your patient's room, at their bedside. Is an alarm constantly going off? Is their IV not running no matter what you do? Is some other piece of equipment not functioning as it should? So many times, the Nurse is so intent (and sometimes perplexed) on the resolution of these issues that she forgets her "face" as well as the words coming out of her mouth as she is focused on the challenge.

The patient and/or their family want to feel that you are capable of solving **any** problem. Do not simply walk out of the room without offering an explanation—especially when the issue is **clearly** still not resolved. These scenarios require closure in the eyes of the patient. Your failure in this regard will leave them feeling uneasy and uncertain about your ability to respond to other issues and needs.

You must never forget the concept that (essentially) you are on stage every time you enter your patient's room. They and/or their family will be looking for clues on your face, signs in what you say and do, and will in turn "judge" how things are going through your interactions and what is accomplished. If you look like you have no idea what you are doing, through your inadvertent commentary, or by the puzzled look on your face, then that is **exactly** what they will perceive. And, you could very well be the sharpest tool in the shed, but you will have just shot yourself in the foot!

Essentially, the fundamental element in your success as a Great Nurse is the professional therapeutic and caring relationship that you establish (*AND* maintain) with your patient. The only knowledge they may (or will) have of you and your hospital is through the words and actions of those who enter the room, in addition to outcomes achieved (or not). Certainly, there may be other factors that inhibit global patient satisfaction; but, a truly *GREAT* Nurse can do much to overcome those impediments through excellent care and sincere compassion. Do not underestimate your power in that regard! You **can** be the dealmaker, but also the deal***breaker***.

One final recommendation is to say goodbye at the end of your shift. Tell them it was a pleasure caring for them (although it might not have been), when you will be on again, *AND* that you hope to have another opportunity to be their Nurse. Whether you realize it or not, they will remember **you** long after you are gone—even if you do **not**. Close the loop and complete your interaction on a cheerful and gracious note.

Do you not say farewell to a guest when they have been to your home? The fact that you are the one leaving should not change that common courtesy. It will leave them with a good impression, acknowledges them as a human being, and it just feels right to say "Good Day" and "Good Night". You never know, they may just want to thank you for taking such good care of them during your shift. If you follow the recommendation from Step Three for Bedside Report with Walking Rounds, this is a perfect time for that transition as you introduce the oncoming Nurse who is about to assume their care.

"Apprehension, uncertainty, waiting, expectation, fear of surprise, do a patient more harm than any exertion."

Florence Nightingale
Notes on Nursing, 1859

Step Twelve
When in doubt, call the Doctor.

Just as you are responsible for all aspects of the Nursing Care of your patients—including care provided by the Nursing Assistant or Tech operating under your Nursing License, at your direction, and with your supervision—so too is the Attending Physician ultimately responsible for all Medical Care provided to the patient. If you work in a teaching facility and deal with Residents and Interns, it is expected that you will follow the appropriate protocols for reporting negative findings and/or obtaining orders. However, *NEVER* hesitate to call the Attending Physician to:

- Report a change in patient status (this is actually a firm expectation/not optional, and should be policy/practice-driven)
- Discuss orders from a Resident or Intern that just do **not** seem appropriate, especially when attempts to clarify or modify the orders have failed (P. S. It is a good idea to bring it to their attention when they give you the order because a smart Intern or new Resident will quickly learn that an experienced Nurse usually knows more about many things than he does himself.)
- Report a serious patient complaint or concern (**No** Physician likes to walk in to a patient's room unprepared.)
- Advocate for the patient in some other way

This applies to the middle of the night, just as the middle of the day.

Always remember, it is the patient who comes first, no matter what. If you are having a problem with a particular Resident or Intern, talk to your Manager and be prepared to speak to the appropriate Chief, Fellow, Physician Liaison, or whoever is responsible for that *Service*. If the problem is with an Attending, bring that to the attention of your Manager as well.

It is more than appropriate for an issue with an MD to be presented to the Medical Director or Chairman of the Department—or to the Chief of Staff, if necessary. No one is above scrutiny when it comes to patient care. Just be sure to follow the Chain of Command and never do anything without your Manager's direction or approval. And—do not forget to document what you have done. If you are not sure what is appropriate to include in the patient's medical record, seek guidance—but cover yourself **and** the patient.

In Summary

Clearly, these Steps represent closing loops, connecting dots, drawing lines, and many other methods for ensuring complete and comprehensive care and communication. They are NOT about loose ends, uncertain answers, incomplete actions, or indecisive approaches. Excellent Nursing Care is about full circles in which you as the Nurse have your patient protected in the center while you cover the perimeter of care for all other *Disciplines* and departments. You are the conduit through which all others must pass. You are the gatekeeper, the filter, the guard, the protector, *AND* the lightening rod.

Nursing is an awesome responsibility. Yet, it is also a gift that is reciprocal *IF* you are smart enough to realize its wonder. When done right, your patients will give you more than you will **ever** give them—and what you give them is (and should be) *A LOT*. It is that amazing human connection not readily a component of most other professions. Never take it for granted. As a Nurse, you often hold someone's life in your hands and have the ability to change it forever. Likewise, it may just as well change yours if you are open to receive.

Even with the professional boundaries that **should** and **do** exist, Nursing can break down a multitude of barriers for the benefit of our patients. Those benefits include both physical and emotional health, as well as spiritual well-being. Nursing offers a unique and rare opportunity to blend Science with Art in the care of one or more human lives. The added professional and personal reward is that of seeing immediate results from actions taken—along with the feeling of instant pride and satisfaction for a job well done. Few other professions can stake that claim. But again, success is measured by effective results and optimal outcomes—all of which depend on an efficient, consistent, and systematic process. Therein you will discover the essence of these Steps.

"It may seem a strange principle to enunciate as the very first requirement in a Hospital that it should do the sick no harm."

Florence Nightingale
Notes on Hospitals, 1863

"101 Little Pearls of Wisdom"
Otherwise known as
THE ABSOLUTELY MUST DO LIST

On Nursing Etiquette and Being a Good Citizen

Pearl #1:
Smile and be cheerful. Your "face" is your first tool when establishing a therapeutic relationship with your patient and/or their family. Typically—your "look", your eye contact, the tone of your voice, and your ability to confidently engage and form that immediate bond (uniquely characteristic of the Nursing profession) are among the many factors that make the difference in your success or failure as a Great Bedside Nurse. Never underestimate the power of a simple smile and a confident upbeat (but genuine) demeanor!

Pearl #2:
Address your patient by name and let them know what to call you. If you have a "white board" (most often a dry erase board) for recording the names of the team and/or other information, *USE IT*! Keep it up to date. Nothing is more disconcerting to a patient and/or family than being admitted to a room in the hospital only to see that the date is not current and the list of caregivers does not reflect anyone currently on duty—yet obviously, someone was just discharged from the room. This small degree of neglect can make them question what else may be overlooked when you are unable to get even the simplest detail correct, such as the current date. This is one of those "no-brainers". Make every effort not to blow it!

Pearl #3:
Let your patients and their families know what your role is in their care, as well as that of others working on your shift, such as a Nursing Assistant or Tech. More often than not, patients think the Assistant is actually the Nurse. You should wonder why and take immediate action to correct that frequent misperception. Many hospitals have resorted to color-coded uniforms to help in this matter, but it is best to proudly state that you are the Nurse, and you might even let them know just how long you have been a Nurse and how long you have been working at your facility. This sends a huge message of competence, as well as a strong commitment to your chosen profession, and potentially to your workplace (in the case of significant longevity).

Pearl #4:
Treat your patients as you would want to be treated. The Golden Rule applies to your patients, just as it does to your coworkers. Imagine how you would want someone to treat your mother, father, spouse, or child. If you work from that premise, you will never go wrong.

Pearl #5:
Take the time to talk to your patients. Know who they are. Sit down for a few minutes (if at all possible) and let them feel they have your full attention. You would be surprised at how well patients perceive a Nurse who actually sits down to speak with them. It helps to solidify that same therapeutic relationship initiated with Pearl of Wisdom #1—based on trust, compassion, and respect. If you are ever lucky enough to work with a Physician who makes time for this simple approach, you will see first-hand just how effective this technique can be. Patients very often trust Physicians with "a great bedside manner", without ever knowing anything at all regarding their base of knowledge and/or their technical skill. We as Nurses know these qualities can often be mutually exclusive, and at times inversely proportional (especially among Surgeons), but the patient typically has not a clue.

Pearl#6:
Know where things are in your hospital and be prepared to give directions to visitors who ask. It is always preferable to escort them to their destination, if you have the time. If not, attempt to find someone who can help out in that regard. Do not leave patients, family members, and/or other visitors to wander about; it is unsafe and can leave them bewildered and frustrated. Neither feeling is a desirable outcome.

Pearl #7:
Make contacts in other departments; they will help you when you need it. If you work a regular shift, you will quickly learn who your peers are in other areas. Get to know them by name. Nothing else facilitates problem resolution quite like calling upon someone you know and with whom you share an easy rapport. You might be surprised how willing they may be to go the extra mile to help you resolve an urgent issue with patient care, even when they themselves are "slammed". These connections can become invaluable over time; cultivate them!

Pearl #8:
NEVER ignore someone who comes to the desk. Stop what you are doing as quickly as possible. Greet them politely, and ask how you might assist them. If

their need is greater than you can manage at that particular moment, find someone who does have the time, but do *NOT* leave them hanging.

Pearl #9:

If you tell a patient you will be back, then *BE BACK*! The minute you say you will return to your patient's room, either they and/or their family begin to watch the clock. Even if you do get tied up by some urgent or critical issue, pop your head in the door and let them know you have not forgotten them, or find someone else to tell them and/or take care of their needs. You will save yourself multiple rings of the call bell if you simply keep your commitments to your patients.

Pearl#10:

If you see someone who looks out of place, ask politely who they are. Do not be afraid to ask for an ID, or to call hospital Security. Hospitals sometimes vary widely on their practices related to visitors. Be certain you know your own hospital's policy and do not hesitate to seek help if something does not feel right. No one who does not have a reason to be on your unit should be lingering about; they should somehow be connected to one of the patients, not simply loitering.

Pearl#11:

If you drop something, pick it up. The Housekeeper has enough to do. Be respectful of *EVERY* member of the team. Pitch in when needed and be certain to empty trash between patients, especially in the Emergency Department. Likewise, learn what goes into the red Biohazard bags and be compliant with those restrictions. There are regulations which (when not followed) can have a huge impact on your hospital, in terms of fines and penalties. Be especially careful about "sharps" (needles and other sharp instruments), body fluids, and/or infectious/hazardous materials. Follow your hospital's policies regarding their disposal and *ALWAYS* be mindful of the next person who will need to handle the bag, i.e. most often the Housekeeper. Protect them from inadvertent injury by "doing the right thing" when working with such items.

Pearl#12:

Never "talk over" your patients with a coworker about your personal or professional business. This includes patients who are unresponsive. You would be surprised by what they may hear and remember once consciousness is regained. It is disrespectful and inappropriate.

Pearl#13:
Also, *NEVER* talk to one patient about another. If it is imperative to give directions to a coworker regarding one patient in front of another, use a generic identifier—and do so in a whisper. Even laypeople are aware of Privacy Regulations, which typically fall under the umbrella known as HIPAA, the Health Insurance Portability and Accountability Act of 1996. Learn the specifics of how this affects you in your practice, as the implications are many, and extend far beyond just talking to one patient about another, or reading the Chart of a patient for whom you are *NOT* caring. Most hospitals require annual education about this and other related topics within what is often known as their Code of Conduct—essentially all those items that pertain to business ethics, and which are mandated by the various regulatory and accrediting bodies at both the Federal and State levels.

Pearl#14:
Learn a second language, or at least the important phrases. It shows you care and have some slight concept of *Cultural Diversity*. Never speak in another language in front of a patient and/or their family unless it is for the purpose of interpreting in relation to some aspect of their particular care—and **only** if you have been officially certified as a Medical Interpreter within your hospital. Likewise, you should never have children or family members serve as the Medical Interpreter for your patient, unless it is a specific request. However, your hospital will undoubtedly have a policy pertaining to this process. Know it and follow the rules and be certain to document all actions related to ensuring full understanding in the patient's own language and/or when dealing with hearing and/or vision-impaired patients. This is another area of critical importance when caring for patients in any setting along the continuum of healthcare, and could have a critical impact on their well-being should you miss key information regarding their symptoms, condition, and/or their understanding of follow-up and/or home care. Your hospital should provide resources by one or more of many means—interpreter phones, live 2-way video, 800 numbers, in-house and/or on-call approved Interpreters, etc.

Pearl#15:
Do not antagonize the *Nursing Supervisor*. She can make or break your day, evening, or night. Trust that she knows the big picture and is not just trying to make your life miserable. Work with her and show her respect. She is most likely having a rough shift too.

Pearl#16:
If you have a problem with an individual coworker, speak to them yourself—if at all possible. If you feel uncomfortable—or you do and it cannot be resolved—seek

assistance from your Manager or the Nursing Supervisor. Do not hesitate to tactfully confront someone who is not doing their job, or is in some way not providing excellent patient care. Be respectful, but do not run away from a problem. Unchecked, the behavior will continue and someone will be harmed.

Pearl #17:
If you have a problem with a process, bring it to the attention of your Manager. Be vocal about what is *NOT* working and be thinking about a solution. Do not be known as a complainer, but neither should you ignore a system that is broken and/or prevents you from doing your best.

Pearl#18:
Go to your Manager with more than just issues about your schedule and/or your paycheck. Show your commitment to patient care. Get involved with activities on your unit and make a difference. Be a good employee *AND* a Team Player.

Pearl#19:
Be a role model to new Nurses. It is up to each of us to lead the way, set an example, and keep our profession alive and vibrant with "new blood". Be enthusiastic—especially with Nursing Students. Do not forget that you were once as naïve as they are now. Believe it or not, you did not spring from the womb as an Expert Nurse.

Pearl#20:
If you are "pulled/floated" to another unit to help out, do not make everyone miserable. Do what you can, but let them know your limitations, especially if it is a specialty area. Ask questions—or for help if you need it. You never know when someone from the same floor may be pulled to your area. Do not make enemies. Build bridges.

Pearl#21:
Do not "call out sick" unless you absolutely cannot walk or stay out of the bathroom. A stuffy nose is no reason to leave your coworkers short. Be a big girl, and hang tough. Of course, if you are contagious…stay home. Act responsibly! Know your hospital's policy regarding Absenteeism and Tardiness. Follow the rules!

Pearl#22:
Be nice to the "Pink Ladies" (or the "Gents in Red"), i.e. the Hospital Volunteers. They deserve your respect and appreciation. In many hospitals, they play an

invaluable role in facilitating flow and communication for patients and their families, as well as those functions that do not require a clinician. Without them, it would be all yours to do. Get to know them by name and show your gratitude for the tremendous contribution they make on their OWN time! Likewise, they are most often involved in a variety of fund-raising activities that benefit the hospital through endowments for many items such as new programs, scholarships, equipment, etc. And typically, they are the folks manning the Gift Shop in the Lobby.

On the Fundamentals of Safe and Effective Nursing Practice

Pearl#23:
Make Hourly Rounds to reassess your patients and their needs. If you cannot get away from a critical situation, ask another Nurse to make rounds for you. Also, depending on your hospital's documentation system, you may have a feature by which you can check-off this fundamental responsibility; however, this can become rote and should actually be individualized to each patient, in terms of what is reflected in your notation. A much better habit is to document frequently regarding *ALL* care provided. This presents a more comprehensive record that better reflects events as they transpired, and will undoubtedly be patient-specific— leaving no room for doubt as to whether or not you actually made the rounds, or just checked a box to demonstrate compliance. Of course, inherent in this approach is that you do make frequent (Hourly, at a minimum) rounds on your patients to assess, reassess, and tend to their needs. If not, you are clearly missing the boat!

Pearl#24:
Know the results of your patients' lab work. Check for those results at the start of your shift and/or as needed, not when questioned by the Physician. This is directly related to Step Three: Know what you are supposed to know. Diagnostic results of all types fall within that category. This is how you learn many fundamentals related to pathophysiology, and by which you gradually gain a much greater understanding of various disease processes, the interrelatedness of many co-morbidities, as well as common complications that occur in the course of either recovery or continued decline.

Pearl#25:
Medicate with PRN medications early and/or on time. Do not wait for your patient to ask. Begin to assess their pain and offer the Medication a half-hour before the PRN is due, and continue to assess and offer every half-hour thereafter. Explain to

your patient the rationale behind Pain Management. This implies that you understand it yourself—as you should.

Pearl#26:
Check the *Crash Cart* yourself on a regular basis, even if it is an assigned task. The reason is (or should be) obvious. The only way you will gain any level of comfort in knowing where to quickly locate items in an actual emergency is by taking the time to memorize their location when you have a few moments of spare time. And, the fact is, there is *ALWAYS* spare time in the course of any shift, *IF* you are organized and follow your System.

Pearl#27:
In an emergency, remember the *ABCs* (now known as CAB). They really do work. And do not forget a backboard. Chest compressions during CPR are ineffective when performed on a soft surface.

Pearl#28:
Get your patients out of bed for meals—whenever possible—but make sure you have an Order to do so. Mobility does wonders for circulation, strength, endurance, *AND* digestion.

Pearl#29:
Know your patient's *I&O*. Fluid and electrolyte imbalances are critical to know and understand, along with the mechanics of whether or not a tube or drain is working as it should. If you have an Assistant or Tech who helps with this task, make sure they know how to accurately record those measurements. Discovering that a patient has had no urine output for your entire shift—or a chest tube that should be draining has had nothing out and the patient is now short of breath— should not come to your attention when an MD is standing in front of you asking for that information. It only takes a minute to check on these things as you spend time in your patients' rooms, so make the time and take note. Be on top of those critical elements in your patient's assessment!

Pearl#30:
Make one last Round before the end of your shift to ensure that all of your patients and their rooms are in the condition in which you would like to receive them. The Golden Rule—one more time, not to mention Patient Safety.

Pearl#31:
Always check all your Charts one last time before you leave. Orders have a way of being missed, no matter how diligent you are.

Pearl#32:
Keep your IV lines straight, especially in the ICU setting. Take the time to carefully separate, label, and secure them—if necessary. Sometimes the "old-fashioned" tricks like using a *Tongue Blade* stand the test of time. Label your *Pumps* but be sure to keep up with any changes as the shift goes on. Nothing is more distressing (or dangerous) than *Precipitating* a line during a *Code* because you failed to make clear what solution or Medication was running into which line.

On Taking Care of Yourself

Pearl#33:
Take a break for meals or coffee—or just to clear your head. If at all possible, get away from the unit for that period of time. Do not eat or have drinks in patient care areas. There are regulations related to this for what should be obvious reasons—namely, infection control—not to mention it simply looks unprofessional as patients and family members are passing through the halls.

Pearl#34:
Do not forget to empty *YOUR* bladder and maintain *YOUR* fluid intake. You cannot think clearly with a full bladder, and dehydration clouds the mind. Nurses are notorious for taking care of everyone except themselves. Try to avoid that bad habit, and/or break it if already guilty. We are often our own worst enemies when it comes to our own health and well-being. Not to mention, we typically make the worst patients!

Pearl#35:
NEVER run to a Code. Walk swiftly and take those few moments to prepare yourself mentally for what will need to be done. Whoever called the Code is already there to get things started, so there is no need to run. You literally "run" the risk of falling, plus you will be out of breath and less able to think clearly once you get there. You need **your** oxygen too.

Pearl#36:
Do not be intimidated by so-called "difficult" Physicians. Being called tenacious can actually be a great compliment. Advocate for your patients, bring concerns to the attention of the MD, and ask questions for the sake of learning something new.

You should **expect** professional collaboration with your Physicians, so do not hesitate to engage them in academic discussions at an appropriate time as they are rounding on your unit.

Pearl#37:
If you are overwhelmed by an assignment—or if it seems "unfair"—never hesitate to speak with the *Charge Nurse*. If that fails to resolve the situation, call your Manager or the Nursing Supervisor. Never walk away from your job or your patients, but do put someone in authority on notice if you are truly in an unsafe situation—due either to volume, intensity, acuity, and/or lack of experience on your part. Once your shift is over, take the time to record exactly what happened for your own records (*NOT* in the patients' Charts). Share your concerns with your direct supervisor, if not already discussed with her at the time. Utilize the Chain of Command as necessary.

Remember there are always occasions when things are crazy, such as when a coworker calls out sick and there is no replacement. Do not be the one who always threatens about jeopardy to her Nursing License, but neither should you tolerate consistently unsafe patient assignments. If this is the way of life in your hospital with no change in sight, you may need to consider whether or not you are willing to participate in providing **that** particular Standard of Care. There may be no other recourse but to look for employment elsewhere. Just be sure it is not simply a transient situation that will improve with upcoming changes in staffing. Also, be sure you have accepted the fact that Nursing is ***Hard Work***. There is rarely an "easy" shift in the hospital setting, so be certain your expectations are realistic.

Pearl#38:
Depending on your personal experience and values, facing the pain, suffering, and even the death of your patients can be one of the greatest challenges in your daily practice. While there is a certain distance that must be maintained to be therapeutic, *NEVER* believe you cannot (or should not) cry with your patients and/or their families. You are human. When the day comes that you no longer feel moved to tears by **any**one's loss or suffering, it is time to get out. However—if grief from working in an area where you are constantly faced with a high degree of emotional stress begins to cloud your thoughts and decision-making, seek help. It may be time for a change. That is perfectly alright. Do not be ashamed to admit to a bit of *Burnout*. It happens to all of us at one time or another in our careers. The important thing is to realize it, and make a decision to take care of yourself **and** your patients.

Pearl#39:
Take care of your Back! Proper *Body Mechanics* is a must, no matter how young you are, or how strong you may be. Many a Back Injury has ended or altered the career of a Nurse who disregarded this simple step. If you do sustain a work-related injury of this or any other type, immediately report the event to your direct supervisor and follow all hospital policies pertaining to such circumstances. Typically, there are strict guidelines and timelines in these matters that will protect your rights as a worker. Failure to do so may result in serious consequences related to much-needed benefits should you lose time from work and/or no longer be able to work in the same capacity.

On Teamwork and Camaraderie

Pearl#40:
ALWAYS work as a team with your peers and subordinates. *NO ONE* is above giving a bath or toileting a patient. If you work in pairs, you will get it done faster and just might enjoy what you are doing a little bit more. Your patients will usually appreciate the timely extra attention.

Pearl#41:
Before you sit yourself down to Chart or go on a break, be sure to ask your peers if they need any help. The best motto to have as a Team is, "if one sits, we all sit". Take note—if you are the only one sitting, while air currents from your peers rushing around are blowing the hair on your head, the thought should cross your mind that perhaps someone else needs your help. Think about it!

Pearl#42:
Never leave the unit without giving a brief Report to a fellow Nurse and being assured that she will cover while you are gone. If you want her to cover for you again, do not leave your patients in pain or with IVs running dry. Failure to do so could be considered as abandonment!

Pearl#43:
Eat, drink, and be merry with the folks on your shift. The team that plays together usually works well together when the going gets tough. Take time to celebrate and know one another. Patients like to see that their caregivers care for one another—as much as for the patients themselves.

Pearl#44:
Communicate, communicate, and communicate! It really **is** as simple as that.

On Common Sense

Pearl#45:

Do not **insist** on reorienting a seriously confused and/or agitated patient. They probably do not *REALLY* need to know the day and date—nor who is the current President—while they are acutely impaired. You will just make them more out of control and yourself crazy by perseverating in your attempts to reorient them. If they give the wrong answer twice, you have yours—they are *NOT* oriented. Forcing the issue will be of no use.

Pearl#46:

Ambulate your patients in the hall—especially your surgical patients—but do not forget to unplug the IV pump from the wall AND disconnect their *Anti-embolic Stockings*. **And**, before you get them up, make certain you have an Order for them to Ambulate.

Pearl#47:

NEVER leave a fresh *Post-op* patient receiving frequent pain medicine (especially with a Pump) alone in the bathroom. If possible, have them use a bedpan or a bedside commode the first time or two—again, do not overlook the need for an Order for them to be out of bed in the first place. Reason A: they may be dizzy or sedated from the Medicine; Reason B: the act of "bearing down" while on the toilet can cause a VasoVagal Response (stimulation of the Vagus Nerve) that can drop their blood pressure and further escalate any sedation or dizziness, which may then cause Syncope (fainting), such that they "fall out" on the floor. Awkward as it may seem, if you are taking them into the bathroom, stand outside the door and *LISTEN*, to ensure their safety. Be certain they know how to pull the emergency cord, if needed. This is one of those times when you must remember that **you** are the professional who knows what is best for the patient, and may need to convince them that your standing guard is for their safety—i.e. the "Art" of Nursing.

Pearl#48:

Provide a fresh supply of water throughout the day, as long as there is no fluid restriction on your patient. You get thirsty and so do they. It is a good idea to ask if they want ice—or not. You would be surprised how many do *NOT* want ice, or only want ice and no water. Also, never forget to take their water away and communicate their status if they are NPO.

Pearl#49:
Prepare your patient for each meal. Wash their face and hands. Clear the overbed table. Sit them up. Put a towel over their chest. When they have finished, take the tray away promptly. No one who is sick wants to smell or look at a plate of half-eaten food. Likewise, assist them with opening cartons and containers and never leave hot liquids with children, the elderly, or patients with any degree of neurologic/neuromuscular/neurovascular deficit or impairment, and/or any degree of psychiatric/psychological disability without **first** assessing their capacity to manage safely on their own. No patient should leave the hospital with a burn related to an accident from spilling scalding liquid on himself or herself!

Pearl#50:
Do not forget to comb and brush their hair. And, hair can/should be washed in the hospital. It is not Rocket Science. Make the time to do it!

Pearl#51:
Mouth Care. That says it all! This applies to patient care in *ALL* clinical settings, and especially in the ICU where poor oral hygiene **may** actually contribute to what is now commonly known as ventilator-acquired Pneumonia (VAP)—simplistically, a form of pneumonia which develops while the patient is intubated (has a tube into their lungs—orally, nasally, or through a tracheostomy in their neck), and is being maintained on a breathing machine (ventilator).

Pearl#52:
Whenever you get a severely abnormal blood pressure, recheck both arms with a manual cuff *BEFORE* you call the doctor—and use the right size cuff for your patient. Make sure they do not have to urinate or have a BM (both can temporarily raise blood pressure—as opposed to Pearl of Wisdom #47, when they are actually making the effort and it potentially drops). Also, have other data available for the MD if you do have to call—such as their other Vital Signs, I&O, any nausea or headache, or other negative findings appropriate to whether it is high or low. Doctors do not like to be put on hold for you to gather pertinent information.

Pearl#53:
Keep your IVs *Patent* and running. Tape them securely. Check the site. Other than the obvious (i.e. injury and/or liability), an IV *Infiltration* is a *HUGE* "dis-satisfier" for a patient and/or a family. Likewise, if the site is lost and you must start a new one, discard the old bag and tubing. Do not potentiate the risk for line sepsis (infection) by using an old setup.

Pearl#54:
Make sure the oxygen is *ON*, not just "on" your patient. Be sure it is in their nose, not just blowing onto their cheek—also, that it is not connected to the Medical Air. It happens!

Pearl#55:
Do not trip over your patient's *Chest Tube*. That should create a clear visual for you with no further need of explanation! The same applies to stethoscopes and other items hanging from your uniform that may snag on the patient's IVs or other critical equipment.

Pearl#56:
Do not test the integrity of the *Foley* balloon by positioning your patient in such a way that the bag is on the opposite side of the bed while the Foley itself is stretched out to the diameter of a rubber band.

Pearl#57:
When they yell "All Clear" in a Code, be sure everyone really is ***ALL CLEAR***. That goes for name tags, stethoscopes, and over-filled pockets that can unknowingly be making contact with the metal bed rails or frame and carry an electric current to you or to someone else.

Pearl#58:
Get your patients ready for bed at night. You brush **your** teeth and wash **your** face at home, do you not? Likewise, the long lost art of giving an *HS* Backrub can do wonders for your patient. Believe it or not, you probably *DO* have the time.

Pearl#59:
Never be afraid to call a Physician in the middle of the night. Just be sure to have all your ducks in a row. Fair is fair. If you are going to wake him up, do not make him wait while you gather information.

Pearl#60:
Make sure your patients receive a bath—even if they decline when first asked. Do not expect an elderly, debilitated, and/or post-op patient to manage the task themselves—and always evaluate a refusal that has been communicated to you by an Assistant or Tech. If they do refuse, offer them another time during your shift—but, get it done. For the short time that a patient is able to be in the hospital nowadays, they deserve to be bathed *AND* to have a clean bed *EVERY* day. The trend of "setting someone up for their bath" typically results in returning to the

room to see a basin of now-cold water and unused soap matched in futility only by the patient's bewildered look as to how they were **ever** to manage the IV tubing through the sleeve of their gown. If you are efficient and work together as a team with your Assistant or Tech, you can knock out a bath and bed change in 20 to 30 minutes. This applies equally to your so-called "self-care" patients. In truth, if they were **truly** "self-care", they would likely not be in the hospital.

Pearl#61:
Do not take your patient's oral temperature immediately after a meal or a drink of something hot or cold. Older Nurses knew this a long time ago. Kudos to those who feel the need to research this "common sense" fact. Temperatures are also usually higher in the evening and typically drop in the wee hours of the morning.

Pearl#62:
No matter how scarce or difficult to find, use pillows for comfort when positioning your patient. Be creative. Nothing causes more pain and/or discomfort than lying in an awkward and unsupported position when you lack the strength or mobility to move yourself. Take a minute and look at your patient from the foot of the bed. It is usually pretty obvious that something is not quite right. Ask them how they feel and take the time to then **get it right**.

Pearl#63:
Ideally, the right time to address *Code Status* with a patient and/or family is **not** as the patient is acutely deteriorating or actively dying. Attempt to develop some comfort with this critical (and sometimes difficult) conversation early on in your career. Acceptance is a process and takes time. Do not overstep your boundaries as a Nurse, but do look for opportunities to broach the subject, if and when it is appropriate to do so. You will be obligated by hospital policy to ask regarding the presence of an *Advance Directive* and/or a *Living Will* at the time of admission, but *End of Life* decisions (and actions) form a continuum. It is always better to discuss these matters sooner, rather than later.

Pearl#64:
When you empty a Foley catheter, be sure to **completely** close the drainage port when done. The smell of old urine is something you will not forget, especially if your patient rooms are carpeted.

Pearl#65:
When inserting a Foley catheter in a female patient and finding the wrong orifice on the first shot, leave that one in place (*IF* the patient can tolerate it), as it will make the next attempt a bit easier and you will hopefully avoid the same mistake.

Pearl#66:
When inserting an IV or drawing blood, hold the skin taut; you are not basting a seam in a skirt. The needle should go straight in, and should not push the skin around by even a millimeter.

Pearl#67:
A fan blowing directly on your patient can help with shortness of breath. Many of your patients with *COPD* may ask for one. Also, make sure they have an overbed table because they *WILL* lean over it as they try to breathe with pursed lips—just as you learned (or should have) in Nursing School! Without one, you may just find them face down on the floor at the side of the bed.

Pearl#68:
If you work the Night Shift, be mindful of the noise you make at the Nurses Station. The volume of night-time noise is one of the most common complaints by patients on a unit. You can enjoy your work *AND* have a good time with your peers without disturbing your patients. This includes loud talking and laughing as much as it does a blaring radio—none of which are acceptable. This applies to the Day Shift, as well.

On Words of Caution

Pearl#69:
When your COPD patient says they cannot breathe, believe them—never assume it is only anxiety. Even if it is, it could quickly decompensate into respiratory distress (each one escalates the other, becoming a vicious cycle), and either condition should be treated. Listen to them—they usually know their disease, and certainly their body, better than you do. If you turn out to be right, then great! Good for you! But, *NEVER* make the mistake of disregarding the early signs of a deteriorating patient. The nouveau term for this is "Failure to Rescue" and has led to the development of the now-standard "Rapid Response Teams" that go by a variety of names, depending on the hospital. The goal is to provide an immediate and comprehensive response to the early warning signs of a decompensating patient. Do not hesitate to use this service if your gut is telling you something is wrong with your patient. Your actions could very well save a life!

Pearl#70:

When *ANY* patient says they have "a little indigestion", take it seriously—do not just give an antacid and forget about it. Take the time to evaluate their symptom as if it were true Chest Pain—especially in women, for whom symptoms are not necessarily "typical", in terms of heart disease. Follow your hospital's protocol, document your actions, and notify the Doctor.

Pearl#71:

Respect your patient's privacy, but guard their safety as well. Be mindful of your patient's visitors and make every effort to ensure that they are welcome by the patient and/or family, whenever possible. Remember that teenagers and young adults pull pranks in the hospital just as they do in the community, and do not always exercise the best judgment about what is safe. Be mindful and check on them frequently.

Pearl#72:

If your patient "just does not look right", go with your gut. No matter what the Physician says, you are probably right. This is a time for tenacity, so be persistent, if things do not improve within a reasonable amount of time. Do what you can to obtain the Physician Orders that you feel are warranted, and if all else fails, do not hesitate to call the Rapid Response Team (see Pearl of Wisdom #69).

Pearl#73:

Be diligent about your patient's routine and post-op *Pulmonary Toilet*. Their *Incentive Spirometer* should not be a toy to take home for the kids or grandkids to play with in the tub. Early mobility (including a "workout" of the lungs) is the key to a speedy (and complication-free) recovery.

Pearl#74:

Be mindful of watching what could be potentially distressing news coverage in the room of a patient who is in some way neurologically-challenged or not fully alert and oriented. Whatever streams into their altered state of consciousness could be misinterpreted and lead to an agitated state due to their inability to fully comprehend and/or respond to what they hear.

Pearl#75:

Try **not** to be shocked if the Vascular Surgeon snaps off a *"Dead Toe"* upon making rounds on his patients. It is pretty gruesome the first time you see it, but it happens. Try not to pass out! It is actually better than finding one in the bed while changing the sheets.

Pearl#76:

Always consider the potential for *Post-Traumatic Stress Syndrome (PTSD)* as a potential cause for agitation or delirium—especially in WWII, Viet Nam or other War Veterans. When they are already confused or agitated, the use of restraints—and even bed rails—can be enough to take them right back in time to that most dreadful experience. Speak with their family and determine any history that could lead to such a response. This applies to victims of domestic violence as well.

Pearl#77:

If your patient *Crashes*, do not leave the bedside. As scary as it might seem, you know them (or should know them) better than anyone else who may respond to the emergency. The only way to overcome your fear is through experience. The more Codes you attend, the more easily you will respond to the next one.

Pearl#78:

Never reposition or re-"tape" an *Endotracheal Tube* by yourself. Few hospitals allow this and some do not even permit the Nurse this responsibility at all. Work with the Respiratory Therapist or another Nurse to complete this task. It *ALWAYS* takes more than one set of hands to do it safely.

Pearl#79:

Know if your male patients are circumcised or not. If not—"manage" their foreskin. If you have never seen a male patient suffer with a foreskin that was left retracted, consider yourself and your male patients as having been lucky. Do not shy away from this important part of your Nursing Assessment. Failure to do so can represent a Urologic emergency, not to mention undue pain and suffering, for your patient. And—*DO* ensure that **proper** bathing is provided for all your male patients, especially those who are *NOT* circumcised.

Pearl#80:

Along those same lines, do not be timid when inserting a Foley catheter into a male patient. It (the penis) is not a dirty tissue to be picked up with two fingers. Improper technique can cause severe damage with so much bleeding and edema that insertion could become difficult—if not impossible—without the use of a special catheter, and possibly only by the MD—as well as the potential for needing an otherwise unnecessary Urology Consult.

Pearl#81:

Never disregard the signs that a coworker might be impaired. The behavior is usually obvious in terms of how they utilize ordered Narcotics (*Opioids*) for their patients. This includes how often they ask their peers to pull Narcotics (Opioids) for them, how they may frequently need to waste Medication not given—along with a variety of other clues that sooner or later should begin to set off an alarm in your mind. Repeated errors in *Narcotic Counts* that cannot be explained can often be linked to a shift when that particular employee is working. Do not make false accusations, but be astute and protect all concerned if you have reason to believe that something is wrong. Speak with your Manager. Your hospital will undoubtedly have a policy or process related to the management of this scenario. While it is not yours to investigate, it is your responsibility to report a concern. This can equally apply to even routine Medications or non-Narcotics. Be aware of any "cultural" misunderstanding in that regard. The Med Room is not one's personal medicine chest. If you yourself are having an issue, see your own Doctor. Do not consider that you can self-prescribe by utilizing those Medications intended for patients. This is a serious violation of hospital policy and State Board regulations. If caught, you will likely lose your job, your License, or both.

On Silly Little Tidbits and Truths

Pearl#82:
Never underestimate the value of a multi-colored pen and a highlighter in keeping you straight.

Pearl#83:
Always have a pair of gloves in your pocket along with a few alcohol wipes, as well as scissors and a clamp. A roll of tape on your stethoscope is a must, as long as you keep it clean.

Pearl#84:
Read your hospital's *Patient Handbook* (if they still have one printed). You might be surprised by what you can learn, even if you are an old-timer. Likewise, take the time to become familiar with your hospital's web site.

Pearl#85:
If you accept a piece of chocolate from one of your patients, be absolutely certain they have never spilled their urinal inside the box.

Pearl#86:
With Russell Stover chocolates, the Coconut and the Orange Cream are on opposing corners diagonally. The Coconut looks like it has bumps.

Pearl#87:
Discourage your coworker from "giving a bad word cue" to a patient with *Echolalia*.

Pearl#88:
There is a limit to how much pressure you can put on a syringe when you are trying to push meds through a small-bore feeding tube. You will never quite forget the sight of a Multivitamin-based/multiple-crushed Medication slurry dripping from your patient's face as they stare at you in total despair, just after it has popped and squirted all over them.

Pearl#89:
If you have never seen it, you cannot imagine what can come out of the ear of an elderly patient with poor hygiene. Some of these things are big enough to be named and have their own Social Security Number. Earwax is serious business!

Pearl#90:
Always appreciate the healing power of laughter, touch, and silence. There is a place for each of them in your daily work with your patients—**and,** amongst your peers. Know when the time is right for one or the other. Hugs are good too! Human Resources (Personnel) may cringe over hearing the word "hugs" due to the global rise in Sexual Harassment charges; however, therapeutic touch is a valid tool in healthcare that should never be underestimated, nor abandoned. A "hug" is one thing; an "embrace" is something else. Let us not overreact and destroy every basic human response to either joy or suffering.

On the Spiritual Side of Nursing

Pearl#91:
When your patient who is actively dying speaks of seeing those who have gone before—or even if you witness a conversation between your patient and someone "not seen" by you—be still and listen. Do not attempt to insert your presence into their reality, and *DO NOT* deny what they are seeing or hearing by trying to reorient them. You would be surprised by what you might experience if you just provide time, space, and support for their journey.

Pearl#92:
Not everyone can handle Death and Dying, yet some exposure is inevitable almost anywhere you work in Nursing. Even if it is something you would rather avoid, do not burden your coworkers by refusing to participate in End of Life care, especially

when it involves the withdrawal of support—as in a *Terminal Wean*. You may never feel comfortable, but—with time—it **can** become less stressful. While you should never be asked to violate your personal belief system, there are certain aspects of Nursing, and healthcare, which are unavoidable. If you are just considering your career, be sure you have thought through all the possible scenarios. Talk to an experienced Nurse if you have concerns. Be clear that you are making the right choice, so as not to compromise yourself or your patients by your inability or reluctance to act.

Pearl#93:

Likewise, even if Hospice and *Palliative Care* Nursing is not your specialty, learn what you can about End of Life Care. It will cross your path no matter where you work, and so often your patients may be surrounded by Physicians and other team members who have little knowledge, understanding, and/or acceptance of this aspect of healthcare. You can do much to advocate for your patient's physical care, as well as their spiritual comfort. Pain is not **always** rooted in the physiologic disease process. Know something about spiritual or *Existential Pain*. Read what you can or talk to a colleague whose specialty is Hospice. You may be the only support your patient has for addressing ALL of their needs on this final journey. And—you **may** just find it is your true calling.

On Being a New Grad

Pearl#94:

When you start out in Nursing, remain calm. Take your time as best you can. Make an effort to learn from the old-timers. You will be surprised by how far you can progress in *ONE* month, 3 months, 6 months, and a year. One day, the light bulb will go on and you will suddenly realize that you finally "get it". You may also recognize what you did *NOT* get and feel a little bit dumb (or maybe even stupid)—but please, do not beat yourself up, we have **all** been there. The journey from New Graduate to Expert Clinician is real—and takes time.

Pearl#95:

Know your hospital's Policies and Procedures within your first 90 days—or whatever your probationary period may be—as a new employee. You may not know every one of them, but be familiar with all that apply to your area of clinical practice. Trying to learn them before a *Compliance Inspection* or a *Regulatory Survey* is as bad as cramming for an exam in Nursing School. Do *NOT* do it! You will forget everything you learned as soon as it is over.

From a legal standpoint, you need to be following your hospital's policies *AND* performing procedures as described in the manual **every** time you provide that particular form of care for a patient. Failure to do so sets you up for personal liability in the event of a negative outcome. Likewise, you must *NEVER* deviate outside your Scope of Practice. If you have not been trained to perform a particular skill and/or it is not within your *Job Description* or on the *Competency* for your discipline, in your area—*DO NOT DO IT*! You will likely be terminated and could potentially lose your Nursing License, or at the very least be put on probation and/or suspended.

Pearl#96:
Despite the allure of starting out in a high-tech specialty, seriously consider the tremendous value of beginning your career on a Medical and/or Surgical floor. Being a "Floor Nurse" is likely the hardest work in Nursing. However, you will learn organization and time management, as well as the fundamentals of communication and patient care, to a degree not easily captured in what might otherwise be considered an advanced area of practice. Beginning as a generalist allows you to develop a strong foundation which can then support you in **any** clinical area, as your career progresses. When you start out so highly focused and intense, you run the risk of early Burnout. Likewise, it can be much more difficult to transition to a generalist role as a Nurse once you have specialized, without having had the benefit of a broad knowledge base and skill set from the start.

Pearl#97:
Your classes on Leadership in Nursing School cannot prepare you for how to delegate to a Nursing Assistant or Tech with a bad attitude. Bear in mind they should not be working there if that is their normal daily behavior, but—the truth is—no profession is safe from unhappy or disgruntled employees. While you **can** do something to modify their behavior on a more consistent basis **after** the fact—and/or possibly even help them realize that this is **not** the career choice for them— you still need to know how to get through the moment.

The first thing you need to understand is that they are operating under **your** Nursing License. It is your responsibility to assess the patient, to assess their ability to perform the task being delegated, and to be certain it falls within their Scope of Practice or Job Description. Likewise, you must supervise them in performing the task if you have concerns about their ability, or if they are a bit inexperienced. If a "confrontation" is unavoidable, do so *OUTSIDE* of the patient's room—preferably in a private area away from the earshot of patients, families, and/or other employees. However, if you need a witness to your discussion, ask the Charge

Nurse or other senior Nurse to participate. If necessary, call your Manager and/or be sure to inform her as soon as possible. Always write a summary of what happened for your own records—that will be especially important for a repeat offender. If you work on an off-shift, call the Nursing Supervisor for support.

The best way to develop a good working relationship with assistive personnel is to get to know them and treat them with respect. However, you must also hold them accountable for their jobs through clear and direct communication at the start of your shift—and at regular intervals throughout until it is time to go—*AND* the job is done. Try to remember what it would be like if you did not have them to do those tasks. The *Nursing Shortage* and the financial realities of healthcare have brought a multitude of changes to our profession—both good and bad. Without a Nursing Assistant or Tech, it is all yours to *DO*—not just to supervise—so take your role (and theirs) seriously. Show appreciation, as well as understanding—and collaborate!

Pearl#98:
Just like **not** specializing too early in your career, so too should you not take on a leadership role until you are ready. Becoming a Charge Nurse is often the first step, as well as a *Preceptor* to new staff. Those two roles are essential components of having "RN" after your name. While it may not be your strong suit, you should never refuse either of those responsibilities. But—be certain you have the experience and the knowledge to take them on at an appropriate time in your first few years of Nursing. Some new Nurses are ready earlier than others; there is never **one** right time. Talk to your Manager about the expectations regarding when to begin in either role, what training is available (there should be a formalized Competency), the frequency of the commitment, and how it might contribute to your advancement.

Pearl#99:
Do not consider going back to school until you have worked at least a year or two as a Nurse. While you may feel quite confident upon graduation, time makes you smarter, more confident, and much more humble. No matter how many "initials" you have after your name, someone still has to get down and dirty with the patient. You should never climb so high on the ladder that you are not willing to roll up your sleeves or in some way pitch in, to help out. To be a Nurse Practitioner, Administrator, Educator, or Researcher without ever truly having been a Nurse at the bedside is like being a musician without ever having had an instrument on which to have played your notes. It is all theory without validation.

Pearl#100:

Never be afraid to ask for help or assistance. You are not expected to remember everything you learned in school. In fact, you might be surprised by how **different** Reality is from Theory. Not to knock the great *Nursing Theorists*, but ultimately, beds need to be made, baths given, Medications passed, tubes drained, and Notes written. With all of that, it is sometimes difficult to wax philosophically, when ultimately it is most often just about getting it all done on your shift in a timely, efficient, effective, and compassionate manner.

Pearl#101:

No matter what, let your patients and/or their families know that it has been a pleasure caring for them and wish them a speedy recovery. Thank them for using your hospital. Learn early in your career—if it is not what called you in the first place—the tremendous gift of Nursing. To provide care and comfort for another human being in need is perhaps the most noble of all professions. Yet—while what **you** give can be invaluable to a patient and their family—what **they** give in return can likewise not be measured. Always take the time to recognize your patients as the unique individuals they are and acknowledge their fears and concerns, just as you would a member of your own family. Listen to their stories as they can become a rich tapestry from which to draw throughout your years of practice. You may not remember **all** of their names but you will undoubtedly remember their room number and what was special about their situation—*OR* what they taught you through your care of them.

Each one of us carries the memory of a few special patients who—for whatever reason—touched our hearts and souls in a unique and unforgettable way. Never become so caught up in the tasks to be done that you neglect the patient in the bed. You should not be doing things "to" him—but "for" him. Even your patients who might be unconscious can hear and smell, and may very well remember or associate feelings with your voice or scent when they are finally able to wake up and be present with complete awareness. You can do much to alleviate their fears through a never-ending humanistic approach—no matter their level of consciousness. Talk to them as if they were fully aware. Even if they **never** awaken to validate your care, you will have given them a final gift and perhaps eased their journey in some way. Always act as if they hear every word you say, and you will never have cause to doubt yourself. Above all, **love what you do**!

"Live your life while you have it. Life is a splendid gift. There is nothing small about it."

Florence Nightingale

A Word about Ethics

There will always be patients who cause you to examine your own values, morals, and ethics—as well as those of the Physician(s) or others caring for the patient along with you. Perhaps a Physician is not the best and his decisions for the patient are poor, or he never spends more than a fleeting moment in the patient's room and never answers their questions. Perhaps the Physician is being less than realistic with the patient in regard to a *Prognosis* or probable outcome. Perhaps no one is advocating for the patient amidst a difficult family that seemingly does not have the patient's best interests at heart.

The scenarios are many and usually reveal multiple shades of grey. Even the most hopeless clinical cases have emerged from states that were seen as nearly unrecoverable. There is not always **one** right answer. However, there should be a means in any hospital to address these situations through an *Ethics Committee* or *Panel*. These resources should be utilized whenever appropriate. Again, it is imperative to follow the process, and to do so in a timely manner so that a patient's care is optimized and their suffering minimal. It is up to each Nurse to search her intellect, heart, and conscience to do what is right—but to do so within the system. It is *NEVER* appropriate to take matters into your own hands, no matter how desperate a situation may seem. Your Nursing License and the future of your career are at risk if you do.

Still, beyond the more obvious ethical considerations related to Prognosis and Plan of Care, there are occasional scenarios when you must confront the behaviors of individual peers and coworkers. This can feel equally challenging and it may seem easier to turn a blind eye, in hopes that the behavior was nothing more than a one-time occurrence. Likewise, you may think that someone else will (or should) deal with it, especially when you are a new Nurse—or new to a particular unit or work-group.

However, in a department with a dysfunctional culture, such behaviors may be widespread and eventually form a curious dynamic—not unlike a hostage situation. These "bullies" maintain poor practice and/or negative attitudes which can go unchecked in the milieu of a weak management structure. Over time, they undermine the integrity of a Team or work-group by dragging down morale. Likewise, the tendency is to also diminish the Standard of Care due to the overall apathy that typically pervades such an environment. In the long run, those who want to do the right thing remain silent out of fear, frustration, and/or disengagement.

When new to a unit or department in which these behaviors become apparent, it is your responsibility to bring your concerns forward by following the Chain of Command. As with anything in Nursing, you must provide documentation, as Management can never act on hearsay or word-of-mouth. Hopefully, the response will be appropriate and the situation will be resolved. In the event that Management is as much a part of the problem through inaction and/or ineffective leadership, you may face your own personal ethical dilemma as to how far up the ladder you want to pursue your concerns, while still maintaining a healthy work relationship with your boss and your peers. However, in the event of serious acts of negligence in patient care, you carry the responsibility for reporting those events immediately. Your failure to do so could be construed as commission, and you could be held equally responsible in the event of a serious negative outcome for the patient(s).

Turning the tide of poor clinical practice and/or a negative work culture is a monumental task and cannot be done alone. Yet, if you find yourself in that situation—*AND* you want to remain in your job—you will be faced with the decision to act. As difficult as it might be, it is the **only** possible course of action if you wish to continue without being negatively affected and/or put at risk in your Nursing Practice. Even the strongest among us find it challenging to remain positive and do our best under such circumstances. This is one of those times when the assumptions referenced in the Prologue must be in place. Namely, you must have a boss who is fair, direct, knowledgeable, honest, and in whom you trust. Likewise, you must be working in a hospital or healthcare system you can support and which equally supports you. If either of those ingredients is missing, you will again have a decision to make as to how much you can do as an individual within your Scope of Practice to effect change in such a negative work environment.

It would be nice to think that these scenarios are few and far between, but—as in any industry—Nursing is not immune to unhappy or dissatisfied workers. Again, this goes back to the premise that all who enter the profession are clear about their career choice and the area in which they have chosen to practice. Sadly—yet not surprisingly—such is not always the case. For some, it can be remedied with a supportive management structure and selection of the right team members. For a Team that has been together a long time, it may mean the facilitation of desired attrition along with a redefinition of the Mission, Values, and Cultural Ethics of the department—all of which should mirror those of the hospital or healthcare system at large.

Again, this is not the responsibility of one person, nor can one person effect such global change alone. But—on a personal level—you could be faced at some point in your career with just such a choice—to be part of creating a solution, or to walk away and find a new opportunity where you can truly excel in a healthy work environment. It is never easy and always requires serious self-reflection along with a careful assessment of what is happening and why. In fact, you should find yourself again utilizing the Nursing Process to assess, plan, act, and evaluate your circumstances. Based on your evaluation, you will determine a modified plan of action. This may be to stay and work toward a solution, or to cut bait and move on.

The most important thing to consider in any situation in your career is your own personal values and whether or not they are supported at all levels of the organization for which you have chosen to work. You may find that the Team is great but lacks leadership from the management structure. Or, the Manager is great but lacks support from Administration for moving the department forward. In some hospitals and healthcare systems, decision-making is truly driven by patient care outcomes. In others, that distinction is not so clear.

As you evolve in your Nursing career, it is imperative to define your critical dealmakers AND your dealbreakers. As you move about from one opportunity to the next, you can do your best to critically evaluate the ability of **any** organization to meet your professional needs in that regard. However, do not be too hard on yourself if you take a new job only to find—once you are into it for a period of time—that it is not what you expected, or is not "as advertised" in terms of the culture or global work ethic of the Team. This has happened to all of us and will require that critical assessment as to whether or not you can be an instrument of change, or should you just move on and chalk it up to "Lessons Learned".

Ethics in Nursing (and in healthcare) encompasses so many diverse and potentially conflicting elements. This complexity requires each practitioner to be crystal clear about their personal beliefs and morals, and to hold firm to their Integrity—often under extreme circumstances. Likewise, it is imperative to remember that we are all unique and therein may lie some of the conflict. You may not live by the same values as your patient or their family, but you must honor their wishes as long as the Standard of Care is met and there is no harm to the patient.

Likewise, you may not be best friends with your coworkers, but you must find a common ground on which to work together for the good of your patients. It is about communication, understanding, acceptance, and respect. No matter the situation—whether it is patient-specific or related to the culture of a department—

there should always be a process by which to address concerns. It is never the work of one person alone and always requires a team effort. Utilize your resources, keep clear and accurate documentation, and never be afraid to voice your issues or concerns in a professional and responsible manner.

Overall, you should discover that the vast majority of those with whom you work have the patients' best interests at heart. It is often the reality of working within a bureaucracy that gets in the way of doing the right thing. For in truth, a hospital is a business—first and foremost. And—every business is fraught with inefficiencies and human error. The key is to minimize those elements and remain focused on the source of that business—the patient in the bed. That is the challenge which again represents the essence of Nursing—to advocate for the patient and their family to ensure safe care with the best possible clinical outcomes.

This is the awesome power of being a Nurse. Your role is the key to so many results, not only for the patient, but for your department and your hospital, as well. Nursing Care **IS** the work of the hospital. Never forget that. Without Nursing, there would **be** no Patient Care. We are the glue that holds it all together. Embrace your unique contribution. Never let anyone diminish our profession nor our vital contribution to the community.

As you grow in your career, advocate for Nursing just as you advocate for your patients. Recognition of our value is critical to any sort of lasting (and successful) healthcare reform. Our voice has the potential to effect massive change in the interest of patients and their families. Learn early in your career to speak up and be heard. Most of all, be true to yourself and keep close to the reason you became a Nurse—to care for your patients. If that drives your actions and decision-making, you will *NEVER* go wrong.

"Were there none who were discontented with what they have, the world would never reach anything better."

Florence Nightingale

What to do about that really "difficult" patient

There always has been—and always will be—that one patient who literally has the capacity to drive you crazy. Either...

- they ring the call bell every time you walk out of the room and they never know what they were calling for when you return
- or they do not like the food
- or the room is too hot or too cold
- or the TV is too loud or too low
- or the light is too bright or too dark
- or you gave them too much ice, or not enough
- or you waited too long, or came in too soon
- or the call bell does not work and the numbers on the phone are too small
- or the sheets are too rough
- or their roommate is too loud
- and—no matter what you do—they just *NEVER* appear to be satisfied

Those are the difficult patients because usually that is just their natural disposition and the challenge is to *NOT* be intimidated. The key is to persevere in trying to meet their needs by being pleasant, patient, and kind. Over time, your diligence may result in at least some semblance of a smile or a kind word, and they may just open up a little so that you—as their Nurse—can see what it is that drives them to be this way. It **can** be done and it is usually about trust and compassion along **with** genuine caring.

The so-called "crusty old man or woman" can usually be won over, but people are typically so turned away by the behavior that they give up and never try to break through the shell. Occasionally, there will be one with whom you can stop in your tracks, turn to them and say—"I am trying my best to meet your needs but I do not seem to be doing a very good job. What is it that would make you feel satisfied with my care?" That may be just the opportunity they need to see their reflection in your mirror and alter their behavior to a certain extent. But—do not expect miracles.

And, unfortunately, there will always be one or two who just cannot be reached. You will have to accept them as they are, not take it personally, and never lose your patience—or your cool. Bear in mind, these patients most often are *NOT* the ones who will rate you or your care as poor. In fact, you may be surprised with just how highly they do think of you. Their behavior is simply their Modus Operandi. They may actually be quite fond of you and satisfied with your care.

The greater challenge is the patient who has a legitimate complaint because something has not gone as expected and/or an error has occurred. This requires honest and clear communication, whether you were directly involved in the situation or not. You must always utilize the Chain of Command and seek support from your Manager and/or the appropriate personnel from any department involved. If you have a *Patient Representative*, utilize that resource as well.

It is crucial to regain the patient's confidence and trust—and ensure that the remainder of their hospitalization goes as smoothly as possible. These are the patients who will share their negative experiences with family and friends and who will rate you, their care, **and** your hospital as poor. They are the most difficult to turn around once the event has occurred—and rightly so. It is best to get Administration involved immediately so they know you take them **and** their concerns seriously, and are committed to correcting the situation—if not for them—for any patients in the future.

A word of caution—when speaking to a patient or family about an incident that has occurred, never admit blame or find fault. Always speak with someone from your hospital's administration—whether it is your Manager, the Supervisor, or someone else in authority—**before** having any conversation with the patient or family, if possible. Always make sure the Physician is informed, as well.

It is critical for Administration to complete a thorough investigation of what went wrong, and the final explanation to the patient and/or family is not yours to make. Do not provide details prematurely and do not speculate regarding the cause or probable outcome. While you must be honest and ensure the patient's immediate safety, do not take matters into your own hands. Doing so may bring the full liability for what has occurred onto you and your Nursing License. As in Ethics, this is another situation where you must use the system.

"If you knew how unreasonably sick people suffer from reasonable causes of distress, you would take more pains about all these things."

Florence Nightingale
Notes on Nursing, 1859

A Few Final Words

If you allow yourself to be open and get to know who your patients are—not just their name, room number, or Diagnosis—but who they are as people, as human beings—you can immensely enrich your practice as a Nurse, as well as your life.

- o To have an elderly man serenade you with a song that he sang to his sweetheart some 70 years ago on their first date
- o To hear the war stories, and even share the tears of remembrance, with a WWII veteran
- o To acknowledge the pain of a wife losing the love of her life after 50 plus years and an eternity full of memories
- o To share in the joy of birth, no matter how many you have attended
- o To visit on your off-hours a patient for whom you have cared—now connected to life support with hands tied down—who asks to write a note upon seeing you enter the room, and does so just to say "I love you" for having been his Nurse
- o To read to a child whose parents cannot (or will not) come to visit
- o To hold someone's hand and tell them it is alright to leave, as their life is slipping away

These are the **great** moments in Nursing!

Embrace your profession! Sing its praises! It is clearly not for everyone. Be proud that you have chosen to care for other human beings, and never let anyone demean you for your choice—nor ridicule your calling. Just like the commercial for the US Army, we do more before 9 a.m. than most people do all day.

Nursing is very much a sorority (or a fraternity, for all you men brave enough to have joined the ranks). When you meet another Nurse—even one with whom you have never worked—there is an immediate understanding, a natural bond. Just make an *Occupied Bed* together. It is like experiencing a secret code.

Those of us with many years of practice must ensure that our profession not only remains intact, but is revived to its original grace. That is our duty as well as our greatest challenge.

The Last Word

Cell Phones. Texting. Emails. Web-surfing. Social Networks. On-line Dating. What has the world come to?

Back in the day, our only distractions were reading a book or magazine, watching television in a patient's room, listening to the radio, talking at the Nurses Station, and possibly knitting or crocheting.

NONE of these activities are appropriate for the image of Nursing. Period! Ever!

Imagine what this looks like to a seriously ill patient and/or their family. They are in pain, frightened, facing a life-threatening illness, losing a loved one, and/or any number of stressors, and they need *YOUR* care. But, what are *YOU* doing? Are you chatting with a friend online? Are you texting back and forth…oblivious to the call bell that is ringing over and over? Worse yet, are you ignoring it? Are you delaying in obtaining their pain medicine? Or in completing their Discharge so they can return home?

Many hospitals are grappling with the management of these 21st Century issues. One thing is clear, you can be held accountable for negative commentary toward your employer and/or coworkers placed on Social Network sites while you are on duty, especially when using hospital property. **And**, there are cases being won and jobs lost, even when you post such derogatory remarks on your own time and/or via your own computer access. Be clear as to what your hospital's policy is in this regard.

Likewise, you must take care to avoid any HIPAA (privacy) violations when it comes to the patients in your care. Legal actions are being taken in that arena as well. Do not be cavalier in your attitude (or your behavior) in these matters. And, beyond that, if you are so unhappy that you feel compelled to present such a negative image of your workplace and/or your patients or coworkers, reconsider the two essential questions discussed in the Prologue. Do you truly want to be a Nurse, and do you truly know what it is to be a Nurse. Perhaps you do not, and it is time to move on.

In practical terms, cell phones have revolutionized our lives, increasing both safety and convenience on many levels too numerous to mention. However, in the workplace, their use should be restricted. Likewise, the use of other forms of media/technology must also be controlled—as much for the message it sends when seen by patients and/or families, as well as for safety and efficiency. Nurse Leaders and Hospital Administrators should take a hard line in controlling these distractions. They are simply unprofessional and unacceptable behavior in the world of healthcare. None of us are being paid to maintain our social contacts, shop or surf, look for love, and/or entertain ourselves with online videos and soap opera reruns.

For the old-timers among us, this behavior baffles the mind. It is unconscionable that anyone would spend **any** time while on duty in such activities, and even more difficult to believe when it is done blatantly in front of patients, families, visitors, *AND* Management. Even with accounting for generational differences, there are still some hard lines in the sand that should be drawn by Administration via Human Resources policies that *SHOULD* carry significant consequences for non-compliance. Again, many hospitals have already taken on this challenge, but the boundaries are still being tested on both sides.

The bottom line in this matter is Integrity and a return to that age-old Golden Rule. Any one of us in the profession should consider how we would feel if we were the patient, or any member of our family were the one in the bed—what would our reaction be when waiting for pain medicine, or to be assisted to the bathroom, or any number of fundamental needs, only to find that our Nurse was sitting at the desk looking for recipes, watching online videos about a toothless man pond-fishing by hand for turtles, or some other ludicrous and non-work-related activity.

In the instant that a patient and/or family in need is seeking you out and finds that you have become distracted and/or have even forgotten their request, you have just destroyed any trust or respect that may have developed, and will likely have severely damaged your therapeutic relationship. Service Recovery at that point can become virtually impossible. And, so it should be, for such a display of unprofessional and insensitive behavior. While on your break or at a meal, surf/text/chat/whatever…but, when on duty and in the patient care areas, the answer is a definitive *NO*!

"If a patient is cold, if a patient is feverish, if a patient is faint, if he is sick after taking food, if he has a bed-sore, it is generally the fault not of the disease, but of the nursing."

Florence Nightingale
Notes on Nursing, 1859

Epilogue

An insidious evolution has occurred in Nursing over the last few decades. Not only has the face of Nursing changed, but its values, attributes, and abilities as well. The more seasoned among us have sensed this slow transformation over time, but now find ourselves unclear as to exactly what has happened and why. The factors are many:

- The shift to an academic, primarily classroom-based education setting
- The push to professionalism in the form of preparation at the Baccalaureate level for entry into the field—with greater emphasis on higher degrees—and no expectations or requirements for competency or longevity at the bedside prior to proceeding with advanced study
- The shift from hospital-based training to more time spent in Long Term Care and Home Care—and all of it drastically abbreviated in time, intensity, and supervision
- The opportunity for women to enter traditionally "male" careers and thereby forego those that were traditionally "female"—thus altering the availability of potentially more qualified candidates who have chosen to pursue other fields of study previously closed to women
- The influx of an international workforce with all the inherent Cultural Diversity
- The ever-present financial influence, with the advent of *DRGs, Managed Care*, and all that followed—up to, and including *HCAHPS*—all of which has radically altered both the appeal and the popularity of a career in healthcare—and Nursing, in particular—after all, why would a young woman (or man) in the 21st century choose a career of hard physical and emotional work which includes frequent exposure to deadly communicable diseases along with the requirement to work weekends, nights, and holidays—and always with the perpetual mantra of "Do More With Less"
- Finally, the state of Nursing is really reflective of the state of society in general—superficiality and frenzy abound in the media, with the perpetual loss of so-called family values a constant political platform—how can we expect a profession that is founded on the most basic fundamentals of care, compassion, clarity, and coordination to survive intact amidst so many societal deviations?—it is no wonder we are where we are in Nursing

To salvage and revitalize, we will have to take a long hard look at our expectations for ourselves, what we will demand of those wishing to enter the field, **and** the process for education at the entry level on through advancement to the highest degrees. Likewise, we must consider requirements for career paths in terms of demonstrated competency and commitment prior to moving to higher positions in **all** tracts of Nursing—whether Clinical, Administrative, or Academic. Essentially, a massive overhaul of the system that produces Nurses is required which parallels the equally necessary overhaul of the healthcare system in general. Perhaps Nursing can help lead the way and concurrently contribute to the greater cause through responsible political activism within our own professional groups and organizations. Perhaps we can finally dispel the myth—and often times the reality—that we "Eat Our Young". Time will tell.

"Hospitals are only an intermediate stage of civilization, never intended at all even to take in the whole sick population."

Florence Nightingale
Sick-Nursing and Health-Nursing, 1893

Glossary of Terms

Abbreviations—Nursing (and healthcare) has what is essentially a universal dictionary of abbreviations for key words, the purpose of which is to simplify documentation. These are (or should be) learned during your initial training and should be consistent from one area of clinical practice or hospital to the next. Furthermore, due to faulty penmanship with the risk for errors in reading the wide range of handwriting in paper charts, certain regulatory agencies have implemented "unapproved" abbreviations that should no longer be used, due to the dangerous ease in misinterpretation unique to similar notations. Failure to follow these standards can result in citations that damage the record of a hospital or healthcare facility. It is essential that you know the standard related to these abbreviations and follow your hospital's policy in this matter, at *ALL* times.

ABCs—Airway, Breathing, Circulation—the essentials of resuscitation. Now known as the CABs, given recent changes to the Science of First Responder Protocols and the latest developments in Evidence-based Medicine to that end.

Additive—simplistically, something that is added, as in the case of intravenous infusions. (See Infusion)

Advance Directive—typically, a legal document that defines the individual's wishes in the event of a terminal or life-limiting illness. Most often this includes language related to being kept alive by heroic measures and/or can specify certain interventions that should or should not be attempted, such as feeding tubes, mechanical ventilation, intubation, and/or the administration of medications, etc. It does not necessarily have to be prepared by an Attorney, and many hospitals have copies available within an informational booklet to be distributed to patients. It will undoubtedly need to be witnessed and/or possibly notarized. If your patient asks you to witness their signature, you should graciously decline and seek support from your Manager and/or the Nursing Supervisor in this matter to help your patient find the appropriate resource.

Laws on this subject vary from State to State. Make the effort to become familiar with those in your particular State, as well as your hospital's policy. At the very least, you will need to ask regarding the existence of an Advance Directive at the time of admission, obtain a copy if available, and/or document the intent of the Directive in the patient's own words. This is a complex topic in healthcare and there are many components, which can be mutually exclusive in their existence. *BUT*, without all the pieces in place, the patient's wishes might not be honored.

This ranges from an Advance Directive or Living Will to a Durable Do Not Resuscitate Order (DDNR) to a Designated Decision Maker to a Durable Power of Attorney for Healthcare to an order for Do Not Resuscitate while the patient is in the hospital. Likewise, certain states include information related to Organ Donation, etc.

The key element is to be certain you know your patient's wishes **and** to ensure that all necessary orders are in place to honor those wishes, especially in situations where your patient is actively declining and/or there is a real potential for sudden death. Again, this is a huge topic, but there are (or should be) resources within your hospital to help both you and/or your patient/family understand all the implications. Seek them out and become comfortable with the information—**not** to be the expert, but to at least be able to facilitate the discussion at an appropriate time, within your Scope of Practice, should that become necessary. (See Living Will)

Anti-Embolic Stockings—any of a variety of brands of electrical devices delivering air to plastic wraps once they have been applied to the patient's legs—creating alternating pressure to minimize the risk for blood clots due to bedrest and immobility, and/or after anesthesia; they also come in non-mechanical forms such as basic compression stockings which should be applied once the patient has had their legs elevated for a minimum of 15 minutes so as not to trap pooled fluid around the patient's ankles, i.e. do not put them on your patient who has been up walking or sitting with legs dependent for an extended period of time. Commonly referred to as "TED" Stockings, for Thrombo-Embolic Deterrent.

Area of Clinical Practice—a unique focus or specialty within healthcare, such as Medical, Surgical, Critical Care, Post-Anesthesia Care, etc. in which a Nurse might choose to work.

Art and Science—a common reference to the blend of finesse and fact, which are key elements in the practice of Nursing. Much of what we do is scientific and frequently "high-tech"; however, there is an equal balance of grace and subtle influence for the well-being of our patients. A case in point might be the sometimes necessary cajoling that is often required to "coax" a patient to follow certain dietary restrictions, or give up smoking, or otherwise follow a treatment plan which they may be reluctant to do. The "Art" involved in Nursing has to do with knowing your patients, understanding their motivations, and then utilizing that information when in the process of educating or persuading, coaching or facilitating compliance toward a desired outcome. The possibilities are many and represent both the "grey zone" **and** the more colorful aspects of Nursing, while the Science remains more black and white.

Likewise, while the "Science" may change, in terms of the "toys" with which we play, such as a new piece of equipment, a new computer system for recording what we do, etc.—the "Art" and the process (or Steps) for being a Great Nurse remain constant. This is most evident when working in the hospital setting and being asked to "float" to another unit to help out. You may not be an expert with that particular patient population and should never be put in the position of performing a skill for which you have no knowledge or experience (or for which you have *NOT* been signed off); however, the basics of Nursing cross all lines. Any one of us can perform all or at least some pieces of the same fundamentals such as bathing, toileting, repositioning, etc. In that regard, never be one to draw a line in the sand saying that there is no way for you to help a fellow Nurse. There is *ALWAYS* benefit in having an extra pair of hands; just be certain to state your limitations in knowledge and experience—but beyond that, pitch in and go to work!

Assess, Assessment—essentially, the process of performing a complete head to toe physical assessment of the patient at the time of Admission and each shift thereafter, **and** with any change in caregiver or level of care (i.e. a transfer from the "floor" to the ICU). The Initial Nursing Assessment is far more detailed and includes many other prescribed data points, some of which are related to behaviors, abilities, home factors, etc. Step One in the Nursing Process. From this, you form a Nursing Diagnosis, which then leads to your Plan, on which you take action (Act/Implement/Perform an Intervention), and subsequently Evaluate your Results. The outcomes obtained then form the basis of any modifications to the Plan, thus forming the complete cycle of a professional Nursing Practice model. (See Nursing Process)

One additional note regarding the actual physical assessment of your patients—you must **actually** place your stethoscope on their skin to hear lung sounds, heart sounds, and bowel sounds. This means *NOT* through 3 or 4 layers of gowns and bed linens, but directly *ON* the skin and in the appropriate location. What can possibly be heard over top of bone—certainly *NOT* the patient's breath sounds moving in and out! Likewise, you must listen for a full cycle of a heartbeat and a breath sound, and preferably for more than one of each, as in several. You must listen long enough to hear bowel sounds in a patient for whom they may be hypoactive. You actually need to palpate (feel) the skin, the abdomen, the pulses—this means you need to take your time, and be thorough. If you are not comfortable with these skills, seek out a resource; but, whatever you do, do not guess. If you are unsure of what you are seeing, feeling, or hearing, find another Nurse to assess your patient with you. Validate your findings. You may just learn something new and/or teach someone else in the process. A truly Great Nurse develops these Basic Assessment Skills and hones them to an advanced Science, whereby when combined with an extensive base of Knowledge, mixed with Critical Thinking, and added to a strong foundation of decisive action—she can do much to accurately predict and respond to what is wrong with the patient long before any test or diagnostic procedure. Likewise, your early intervention and notification of the Physician regarding your findings can alter the course of the patients' illness for the better and hopefully expedite their recovery and Discharge from the hospital.

Assistive Device—essentially, anything the patient uses for mobility such as a Cane, Walker, Crutches, or Wheelchair; however, this may also indicate items such as "reachers" and "grabbers", or specially designed shoe horns, etc. There is a wide range of devices that can be adapted to assist with personal care, mobility, and the Activities of Daily Living (ADLs) for the purpose of maintaining independence. This is the primary role of both Occupational Therapy (OT) and Physical Therapy (PT).

Bedsores—the common term for what is actually known as Pressure Ulcers; also known as Decubitus Ulcers; lesions that form essentially from prolonged pressure over a bony prominence, i.e. e.g. typically, the hip, sacrum (tailbone area), elbows, knees, ankles, heels, the back of the head, and even the ears. Their development and progression are dependent on many factors to include immobility, poor nutrition, underlying disease process, moisture, friction with movement, and age. This is a complex topic in healthcare in that the development of these pressure ulcers while in the hospital will adversely impact the rate of financial reimbursement by the government and other insurance agencies.

It is absolutely critical that every patient be assessed from head to toe upon Admission so that any ulcers existing at that time can be appropriately documented—at present, within the first 24 hours, by current regulatory standards. This may (and should) require the assistance of a Wound Ostomy Continence Nurse (WOCN)—previously called an ET (Enterostomal Therapist)—who can assist Nursing staff with the necessary measurements and "staging" that must occur to accurately document the severity of the wound. Without those details, there is no means to track the progress, or the decline. Likewise, the depth and condition of the wound will determine the recommended treatment plan.

Your hospital will (and should) undoubtedly have a protocol addressing this fundamental of Nursing Care. There should be a prescribed assessment scale to measure any/every patient's potential for risk related to the development of these wounds. Likewise, the most basic requirement is for *EVERY* Nurse to examine her patients' skin at the time of Admission. This means direct observation, as in without a gown or bed linens, except for comfort or privacy. It is never acceptable to ask the patient if they have any wounds and let it go at that. You actually must lay eyes on all key places where these wounds can form—essentially, head to toe. No exceptions on this one.

This means you turn your patient from side to side, in a well-lit room—and, seek help to ensure your patient's safety and comfort during this process. Any area of redness must be assessed for the integrity of the skin and Capillary Refill [the return of circulation when pressure is applied to blanche out/whiten the skin—it should return within 2-3 seconds (for adults), meaning normal; if longer than 2-3 seconds, it would be considered delayed—indicative of possible/potential tissue damage]. Again the Science of skin and wound care is extensive. Take the time to learn as much as you can. After all, the Skin is the largest "organ" of the body.

Best Practice—a relatively nouveau term that essentially means the Standard of Care, but in most cases would be considered to include Evidence-based Medicine and/or Nursing. That which brings the best possible outcomes in patient care, and would be identified as such in a court of law. (See Standard of Care)

BM—Bowel Movement.

Hidden Bonus Pearl: when inserting a suppository, only to have it pop back out after multiple attempts, as it begins to melt in your gloved hands such that you anticipate needing a replacement, try again; but, insert the blunt end (counter-intuitive, yes—but it works!). No matter what, you need to insert beyond the external anal sphincter, however in some patients with extreme "tone", this can become a challenge. By inserting the blunt end first in these patients, the body naturally pulls the suppository "in", rather than pushing it "out". Makes sense!

Boards—also known as the State Boards; essentially the State-administered exam through the graduate's respective Board of Nursing that ensures a common and minimally acceptable core of knowledge among those having graduated from accredited Schools of Nursing. "Passing your Boards" is what affords you your Nursing License as a Registered Nurse. The same applies to other levels in Nursing such as a Licensed Practical Nurse or a Nurse Practitioner. Your license is State-specific and must be renewed by paying a fee. Some States require Continuing Education Units (CEUs)/Hours prior to renewal.

Body Mechanics—those techniques designed to avoid unnecessary strain and/or injury when pushing, pulling, lifting, or providing other forms of patient care. The Physical Therapists and your Employee Health Department are good resources in these matters. Use them. Likewise, your hospital may very well have a Competency for this topic, as well as specialized equipment, as they have a vested interest in preventing injuries to their workers (as well as to patients).

Burnout—the phenomenon of overwhelming and incapacitating grief or despair that may occur as a result of chronic exposure to high levels of stress—along with the grief, loss, and suffering of your patients and/or their families; may include other emotions and typically leads to an inability to function effectively.

Care Model—essentially, the design by which care is provided to patients on a unit. This may be what is known as Primary Nursing where one RN has responsibility for an assignment of patients with or without assistance. Another model is known as Team Nursing in which one or more Licensed Nurses have responsibility for a group of patients with or without assistance. The variations are many. This may include Registered Nurses (RNs), Licensed Practical Nurses (LPNs), Nursing Assistants or Techs, and any variety of combinations of Disciplines and skill mixes. (See Model, Model of Care)

Care Plan—multiple meanings, but essentially, what is planned for the patient. May also be referred to as the Plan of Care. Encompasses both Physician Orders and Nursing Actions.

Chain of Command—the hierarchy of Management to Administration that exists in the hospital setting for reporting/addressing issues and/or effecting change.

Charge Nurse—a more senior Nurse responsible for overseeing the activity and care on a unit for a specific shift, often in addition to caring for her own patient assignment. May be referred to as the Resource Nurse or the Team Leader, among other terms.

Chart—that which represents the record of the patient's hospitalization; may be entirely on paper, or a mix of paper and an Electronic (Computerized) Medical Record (EMR). To "chart" means to document or record everything you do in the course of providing care to your patients. Cardinal Rule: if it is not documented (charted), it was not done. Your charting is all you will have to explain actions taken and care provided. It does not matter what you *SAY* you did, only what you **recorded** that you did. In the end, the patient's medical record is the single source of facts in any legal case. Period.

Chart Checks—the process of reviewing all orders in a chart for a defined period of time to ensure that all Physician Orders have been initiated and/or completed.

Charting—the process of documenting defined elements of a patient's hospital stay; that which creates the patient's Medical Record or Chart.

Chest Tube—essentially, a tube inserted through the skin, between the ribs, and into the patient's lung to remove fluid, pus, and/or in the event of a collapsed lung. It is most often connected to a drainage system, with or without suction, and is typically sutured in place and covered by an occlusive dressing.

Clinical Excellence—the provision of first class/top shelf patient care that achieves optimal clinical outcomes. Many hospitals utilize the term "world class" care, which inevitably leaves it open to interpretation and/or ridicule when the care is poor, as if to say, "Which world, the third world?". Better to say *FIRST* class, leaving no room for doubt!

Code—typically, a Cardiopulmonary Arrest; may go by different terms depending on the hospital.

Code Status—also known as Resuscitative or DNR (Do Not Resuscitate) status, i.e. do they want to be resuscitated should their heart stop and/or they stop breathing. Policies vary slightly by hospital, and laws pertaining to the same vary by State. Be sure you know both. (See Advance Directive)

Competency—a defined skill, and the process for ensuring proficiency with that same skill; these are discipline-specific, i.e. the Nurse, the Tech, the Assistant, etc. and vary by department; likewise, there are typically generic hospital-wide competencies that are universal to all disciplines. They may be validated at the time of hire during the orientation process and/or annually (or more often) thereafter. This relates to Scope of Practice and dictates the care you can (or will) provide to the patient, as well as the boundaries for said care which must not be crossed.

As the Nurse caring for the patient, it is your responsibility to know those tasks which can be delegated to Assistants or Techs working under your License. Likewise, you must be certain they are competent to perform those skills independently. If not, you must directly supervise their work. In some areas of clinical practice, their work must be routinely supervised and documented as such to meet regulatory and compliance standards, i.e. e.g. Home Care and Hospice.

Compliance Inspection—the process of ensuring that a hospital or healthcare facility meets defined standards or criteria related to patient care; typically administered through the State's Department of Health; results in the licensure of the organization, which is necessary for the receipt of reimbursement from the government and other funding sources.

Computerized Physician Order Entry—a process by which Physicians directly enter their Orders into a computerized system (Electronic Medical Record), as opposed to writing them on a Physician Order Sheet in a paper Chart, which must then be transcribed and/or entered into a computer system by a second party, such as the Nurse or the Unit Secretary. The only drawback to Physician Order Entry is that other than their Progress Note where they might indicate the planned order— or if they communicate the Order directly to you before or after entry—you must rely on that which spits out of the computer (or appears in an on-screen worklist) as correct and what was intended, as there is no other backup. In many facilities, not all Physicians have equal knowledge of the computer system, and their lack of proficiency may lead to errors. This increases the urgency of your need to know your patients well, and to evaluate the appropriateness of every Order in relation to each individual and their needs.

Consult, Consulting, Consultants—the process of contacting Physician Specialists to participate in the care of a patient. This is in addition to the Attending and/or Admitting Physician. May also apply to other disciplines or areas of professional practice and expertise.

Coordination of Care—the process by which the Nurse manages the care of the patient; this may be within the context of a multidisciplinary team, and should be an active process based on communication and planning. Clearly, every department in the hospital has its own routines and schedules; however, a Great Nurse takes responsibility for facilitating a Plan of Care that best meets the patient's needs. This may require contacting other areas to inquire as to planned interventions, to suggest a different time if and when that is possible (such as with Therapies, when the patient might have better outcomes when not already fatigued from multiple other activities), and/or to facilitate contact with key providers when the family is unexpectedly present (such as with Case Management for the purpose of early Discharge Planning, or the Doctor for discussing the patient's Prognosis).

The possibilities are endless, but essentially, the intent is the same. The Nurse is (or should be) the driver of all patient care on her shift, and should facilitate the plan for the next shift through strong collegial relationships with all other members of the patient's healthcare team. This is another fundamental element that comes with having "RN" after your name. Do not abdicate this basic responsibility! Your patient will suffer and you will be completely ineffective in your role as Patient Advocate.

COPD—Chronic Obstructive Pulmonary Disease, also known as either Chronic Bronchitis or Emphysema.

Crash—when your patient suddenly "goes bad" and becomes acutely compromised, possibly resulting in the need for resuscitation.

Crash Cart—the large rolling cart that is swiftly brought to the patient's room or to some other site of a Code; contains most things needed for resuscitation. Your hospital should have separate carts for adults and pediatric patients. Know the contents of each drawer like the back of your hand!

Critical Thinking—simplistically, the ability to respond to any situation with a complete assessment and appropriate plan of action based on experience and a highly evolved ability for processing all available information in a thorough and systematic manner to achieve the best possible outcome—most often in split-seconds, such as an emergency.

Cultural Diversity—a relatively nouveau concept that has quickly become a requirement, in terms of education and patient care. Essentially, the recognition that both patients and caregivers may come from a variety of cultural backgrounds, affecting perceptions and understanding at both ends of the spectrum—related to values, practices, and beliefs. A key lesson with regard to Cultural Diversity is to never make assumptions, nor assume understanding or meaning. You must always validate and establish a common ground on which to base your care—especially when related to patient and/or family teaching. Without that connection, compliance with the Plan of Care may be virtually impossible. Likewise, you should never be so arrogant as to presume to change deeply held values and beliefs. Be open to viewing life and health from a new and different perspective. It just might make sense (right or wrong) if you are compassionate enough to listen. In turn, it may provide you with an avenue for changing perceptions and thereby improving outcomes.

Current Condition—not exactly a formal technical term, but simply the state of the patient at the moment; their actual physical assessment at the time that information is needed.

Dead Toe—a toe that has been robbed of circulation for so long that it appears like a crusty piece of charcoal which literally breaks off with minimal pressure.

Delegation—the process by which the RN first assesses her patient(s), then determines the availability and competency of any assistive personnel who may participate in the care of that patient, followed by the delegation of select elements of that care, while still retaining accountability for its completion and the evaluation of its outcomes. This requires that the Nurse is knowledgeable as to the Scope of Practice of that individual and has the means to ensure that they have been validated as competent with regard to those specific tasks. This is typically done via the use of a Skills Checklist or some other form of Competency documentation.

A key element in this process is that *NO* discipline, including the RN (experienced or not), should be providing care to the patient for which they have not been validated as being competent. Likewise, it must be covered within their Job Description and/or Scope of Practice. Failure to meet that restriction can/will result in disciplinary action up to and including termination of employment. In some cases, it may be reported to the respective Board, such as the Board of Nursing— potentially resulting in further disciplinary action against your Nursing License. Delegation is complex, and yet on some level still relatively simple. It is governed by the State Board of Nursing and should be completely integrated into any Model of Care, on any unit where the Skill Mix of available or assigned Disciplines mandates that it must occur. Know both the law and your hospital's policies in this matter. (See Board, Competency, Job Description, Scope of Practice)

Diagnosis—that which the Physician has determined to be "what is wrong with" the patient; i.e. the illness or disease process identified through the variety of testing that was performed during a patient's hospitalization, based on symptoms and other objective and/or subjective findings. The Diagnosis may be a temporary condition that will resolve with Medication or other interventions and could therefore be considered Acute—meaning sudden and limited; or, it could be (or become) a Chronic and permanent condition that will require long-term management of its symptoms, with or without flare-ups or exacerbations—meaning that the disease may be worse at times related to certain identifiable triggers or for no apparent reason at all.

Essentially, in practical terms, diseases can be Acute or Chronic *AND* chronically acute or acutely chronic. It is the management of chronic illness that is the most challenging and with which we sometimes have the least success, in terms of outcomes and quality of life. Likewise, it is where we will (and must) undoubtedly focus the majority of our attention in the coming decades within healthcare—not only on its management once present, but more importantly, on its prevention.

Discharge Instructions—a form and a process for closing the loop at the time the patient leaves the hospital. At a minimum, this should include the Discharge Diagnosis, special instructions related to Diet, Activity, and the care of wounds, drains, or other ongoing specialized Nursing Care to continue at home. Likewise, there should be information regarding follow-up medical care and when the patient may return to work or school. In addition, there should be a reconciliation of Medications to be continued or discontinued—along with any prescriptions, when ordered.

Discharge Planning—the process that **should** to begin at the time of Admission, by which data is collected as to the patient's home environment, such that plans can be made for a safe discharge based on the patient's anticipated condition when ready to leave the hospital. This would include care that will be needed, who may be available to provide that care, the physical environment in terms of safety and necessary equipment, and whether or not an alternate care setting might be required permanently, or for a short period of time prior to returning to their pre-admission home. Data is collected within the Nursing Admission Database and should be communicated to all members of the healthcare team. Note: terminology for various forms/documents may vary from one hospital to the next.

In the event of special needs, it is typically necessary to involve Social Work or the Case Manager—depending on your Care Model—so that these issues can be addressed in a comprehensive manner, such as funding sources for alternate care, contact with facilities for bed availability, providing lists of agencies that offer in-home care, etc. All hospitals are required to conduct Interdisciplinary Rounds that include all members of the healthcare team. These may trigger the need for a Discharge Planning Consult or the Nurse may obtain an Order for one at any time, based on her assessment of the patient's needs.

Discipline(s)—typically, this refers to other members of the healthcare team, i.e. e.g. Physical Therapy, Occupational Therapy, Speech Language Pathology, Respiratory Therapy, Social Work/Case Management/Discharge Planner, etc. Ultimately, the Nurse is responsible for coordinating all care of the patient (by definition); however, as discussed there are those who fail to recognize this critical role, thereby abdicating not only their professional accountability, but also their critical influence on effecting optimal patient care outcomes.

Doctors Order Sheet—in a paper Chart, that form where the MD creates Orders for Medical and Nursing Care; typically a multi-part form; that which is checked during the process of Chart Checks. May also be known as the Physician Order Sheet. In the case of Computerized Physician Order Entry (CPOE), this will all be electronically automated, such that Orders print out and/or feed over to other computer systems for various departments within the hospital. However, there must still be a process for validating the accuracy, appropriateness, and completion of Orders. (See Computerized Physician Order Entry)

Documentation—the process of recording all care provided for the patient. (See Charting)

Documentation System—many meanings, but essentially the process by which the Medical Record is created; may be entirely computerized and also known as the Electronic Medical Record, may be entirely on paper, or a combination of both; computerized systems vary by clinical specialty and do not always interface, and/or do not interface well; however, barring any legislative changes, certain 2015 government-mandated regulations should minimize and/or eliminate these discrepancies with system integration. (See Chart)

Dress Code—usually, a policy within a hospital or other healthcare setting that defines (often by Discipline or Job Description) all parameters for how to dress, including the use of jewelry and perfume, as well as such items as hygiene and make-up—including nail care. There are regulations pertaining to the use of nail polish and artificial nails for which violations may result in fines for your hospital and disciplinary action for you. Do not take these matters lightly. You could even be sent home to change clothing should you fail to comply with these expectations.

DRGs—Diagnosis Related Groupings; essentially, a methodology utilized for determining the rate of financial reimbursement.

Echolalia—a condition in which the patient repeats the last word or phrase heard over and over until triggered to say something new.

Edema—swelling.

Electronic Medical Record System—a computerized method for creating and maintaining the Medical Record. (See Chart, Documentation System)

Emergency Department—essentially, the gateway into the hospital for many patients who come to receive care for urgent, emergent, and life-threatening conditions, either by walking in or by being transported via ambulance. The ED, as it is now known (vs. the ER/Emergency Room), has also become an alternative for those patients who lack a Primary Care Physician due to not being insured. As a result, many Emergency Departments are overrun with patients looking for basic care that could best be provided through a Physician's office and or other out-patient service, commonly covered by health insurance. This, in turn, has resulted in long wait times and over-crowding.

What the public must come to realize, and what lawmakers must soon address, is that the Scope of Care provided in the Emergency Department is not intended to meet the needs of the chronic conditions and pain issues for which many of these patients seek service. Likewise, hospitals must structure their operations to manage capacity via efficient inpatient care through utilization of an integrated multidisciplinary approach that facilitates flow, and decreases length of stay, yet not at the expense of desired clinical outcomes, which would only increase readmission rates and thereby perpetuate the cycle of overcrowded EDs.

End of Life—in simple terms, that time period in a patient's life, most often associated with a known terminal illness during which their condition is beginning to decline. This represents another stage in the continuum of care with which many Physicians and Nurses are unfamiliar and/or uncomfortable. Hospice and Palliative Care is a Board Certified specialty in Medicine as well as a Certification in Nursing through the professional organization dedicated to its practice, and is quickly becoming required curriculum in both medical schools and Schools of Nursing. The care provided to a dying patient and his or her family encompasses not only physical needs, but emotional, social, and spiritual as well.

Endotracheal Tube—a tube that passes through the nose or mouth, into the trachea and to the lungs, to provide an airway for use with some form or oxygen, and possibly mechanical ventilation.

Ethics Committee or Panel—a multidisciplinary group that meets regularly and has availability on a 24/7 basis to address ethical dilemmas in patient care; typically, they are not a governing body and cannot mandate policy or practice, rather they **can** make recommendations based on specific information presented by those involved in the care of a particular patient.

Existential Pain—pain with a spiritual and/or psychological origin that may contribute to and/or exacerbate actual physical pain, making the latter more difficult to manage. In fact, Existential Pain may be the most difficult to control.

Fall—a Fall is essentially just that, the patient falls, either from the bed, while ambulating, off the toilet, etc. The Fall may occur while the patient is alone (Unwitnessed), or while you or someone else is present/observes the Fall (Witnessed). It may even be what is called "Assisted", meaning that you or someone else is with the patient as they are beginning to fall, and assistance is given to lower them to the ground or some other surface, in a controlled manner, to minimize the potential for injury.

Actions to be followed after a Fall include the following: ensure the patient's immediate safety by providing a pillow, blanket, and/or positioning for comfort until you have assistance to get the patient up from the ground in a safe manner; immediately assess the patient for any obvious injury; immediately notify the Physician, your Charge Nurse, the Manager and/or the Nursing Supervisor; ensure that any Orders such as X-rays are completed in a timely manner; move the patient back to the bed as quickly as possible, once it has been determined that there are no serious or life-threatening injuries that could be made worse by moving them. Likewise, you must notify the patient's family *AND* you must make a note of the Fall in the patient's Chart.

Your documentation should be clear, concise, factual and non-accusatory as to the possible cause. You must remember that this note could be viewed by an Attorney and/or in a court of law at some later time, so do not make assumptions as to why the patient fell. Your only obligation is to state that the patient fell, what the patient was doing at the time of the Fall, whether or not it was witnessed and/or assisted, what actions were taken immediately after the Fall, if the Physician saw the patient, and/or whether or not Orders were given and completed. Be certain to note your efforts to contact the Physician and obtain Orders, especially if you feel the patient *SHOULD* be evaluated and Orders given.

You must do everything within your Scope of Practice to ensure that the necessary care is provided to the patient, which may mean utilizing your Chain of Command to get things done. Essentially, be tenacious and do not accept "No" for an answer if you believe the patient requires further evaluation and/or intervention to ensure their safety. Finally, you will likely need to complete an Incident Report. This is a computerized and/or written tool used by the hospital's Risk Management department to track such occurrences and to gather additional information that might be needed in the event of legal action by the patient and/or their family. It is also used to track trends across various departments of the hospital that may indicate the need for safety programs and/or specific interventions to minimize the incidence of Falls and/or other unexpected events overall. Follow your hospital's policy in this matter.

Also, when speaking with the family about the event, never make reference to this internal report and *NEVER* assign blame in any way or make any declarations as to who or what may have been the causative factor in the Fall. Simply state what happened and what you and/or others did to ensure the patient's safety after the event. Finally, be certain to pass on this information in Report to the oncoming shift, and take whatever actions are recommended by your hospital's policies to implement ongoing "Fall Precautions" for your patient. This may involve the use of a special arm band, alert magnets on the door frame, a bed alarm, and/or a variety of other safety measures that will (or should) be part of a prescribed program to prevent such occurrences.

Make frequent rounds on your patient following the Fall and reassess for the following at regular intervals: neurologic status, Vital Signs, pain or discomfort and what measures you have taken to relieve said pain, appearance of the skin in the area of contact looking for the development of any bruising, and the status of any wounds or other injury that may have occurred as the result of the Fall. Document all of these activities and assessments in a timely manner, as well as your ongoing measures to ensure that there is no repeat Fall.

It may even be necessary to provide a "Sitter", depending on the condition of the patient and their ability and/or willingness to follow directions. This individual would remain at the patient's bedside, to be immediately available with a direct line of sight to ensure the patient's safety. Sitters may also be utilized in other patient care scenarios such as with Behavioral Health patients who may be suicidal or homicidal. Those cases involve many other safety measures and it may be best to utilize different terminology for the word "Sitter" in that event, in order to distinguish the significantly greater level of awareness that must be present with those kinds of patients. This is a huge topic and you must know both the Standard of Care and your hospital's policies in this matter.

Feeding Tube—any of a variety of tubes that are utilized for the purpose of providing artificial nourishment. They may be passed through the nose into the stomach, or inserted surgically through the skin.

Florence Nightingale—essentially, the founder of modern Nursing. All quotes utilized within this volume are credited where known, in terms of the source book, letter, or essay. A few others commonly attributed to her, and readily found on any search of the internet, cannot be mapped to a specific origin—and, therefore, have no notation to that end.

Foley—a catheter inserted through the urethra and into the bladder to drain urine; held in place by a balloon that is inflated with Normal Saline solution. It may be left in place (indwelling) and attached to a drainage bag, or it may be a one-time "in and out" procedure to empty the bladder for a particular reason, in which case there is no balloon or the balloon is deflated prior to removing the catheter.

Golden Rule—the age-old message, "do unto others as you would have them do unto you". This concept has existed throughout the history of the world and within all religious faiths. While some might argue that the "Platinum Rule" is best (i.e. treat others as **they** would want to be treated), the majority of us understand the concept. Essentially, it is about treating your patients as you would want either yourself or a member of your family to be treated—in terms of care, compassion, respect, understanding, and comfort. Again, this is not Rocket Science. Likewise, this applies to all professional relationships—peers and patients.

Graduate—a plastic container for measuring liquid.

Great Nurse—that one (and hopefully more than one) Nurse who has it all together and makes it appear effortless; the epitome of clinical excellence. (See Clinical Excellence)

Grievance—part of the continuum in the complaint process, and usually the most severe of possible demands by a patient (other than a lawsuit)—in terms of desired action to resolve an issue or negative outcome. Your hospital will likely have strict guidelines and timelines for responding to such matters. Understand your role in facilitating a response; and, better yet, be astute to potential conflicts before they have the chance to escalate to this level. This means, know your patients and determine their satisfaction with (and understanding of) their care.

H&H—Hemoglobin and Hematocrit, a common blood test. Often referred to as the "Blood Count".

Handoff in Care—the transition of Nursing Care from one caregiver to another; requires a detailed report as to the patient's History, Current Condition, and Plan of Care—among other facts. This applies to both Shift Change and to patient movement from one department to another. Some hospitals utilize a "Ticket to Ride" as a tool in this regard which is nothing more than a small form used to convey key pieces of patient information to ensure safety, as when a patient travels to Radiology or some other area for a test or procedures. Likewise, there are even longer forms with a similar intent, such as a "Pre-op Checklist" to be used for a patient going to surgery to ensure that all necessary items have been completed as required by hospital policy. Again, the content material here is extensive. Utilize all resources to be compliant with your hospital's policy and the Standard of Care.

HCAHPS—Hospital Consumer Assessment of Healthcare Providers and Systems, or simplistically, the current reimbursement methodology based on Patient Satisfaction, the driver of which is most often related to elements of Nursing Care.

Health Unit Coordinator (HUC)—the Secretary on a Nursing Unit or Department.

History—the process and the result of the Physician obtaining information about the patient's health throughout their lifespan to date; part of the Medical Model; may be known as the History and/or the History of Present Illness (HPI); the larger process includes the Past Medical History (PMH), Past Surgical History (PSH), Social History (SH), and the Psychiatric History (PH); similar to the process of the Nursing Assessment, but the latter is more holistic in its approach.

Home Care—the business and concept of taking Nursing (and other healthcare) to the patient in their home.

Hospice—a philosophy, a program, and a benefit under most health insurance plans for providing care and support to patients and their families in the presence of a life-limiting illness, through and beyond the time of death.

Hospital Nurse—a Nurse who has chosen to work in an acute care clinical setting in a hospital; the possibilities are varied, in terms of specialties within that context.

HS—Hora Somni (Hour of Sleeping)—At Bedtime.

ICU—Intensive Care Unit.

I&O—Intake and Output, or measuring what the patient takes in by all forms, and what comes out by all means.

Incentive Spirometer—the funny little plastic device with one or more columns for "pushing" up a marker with each Inspiration, thereby helping your patient take deep breaths and fully expand their lungs, especially after surgery. It works! Learn how to use it yourself so that you may properly instruct your patients.

Incident Report—an internal hospital document for the purposes of Risk Management by which unexpected events and/or outcomes are documented. May go by varied names. May be computerized and/or on paper. Remember to **never** make reference in your notes to having completed this report.

Infiltration—when an IV becomes dislodged and fluid seeps into the tissues rather than passing through the vein, such that the area becomes swollen and painful. This requires immediate intervention to provide comfort and to prevent further injury. This can be particularly dangerous with certain IV infusions (or drips) in which a particular additive (or Medication) is toxic to the tissues of the skin. Emergency responses must be immediately implemented to prevent permanent damage and/or disfigurement.

Informed Consent—a form and a process for obtaining the patient's agreement in writing, prior to a procedure, surgery, certain tests, and/or some treatments. This is the sole responsibility of the Physician who must explain what is to be done, the benefits, risks, and any potential for complications or side effects. Know your hospital's policy in this matter. Never deviate from that Standard of Care, and never be timid about reminding the Doctor of his role. Likewise, this must *ALWAYS* be done before, *NOT* after—especially when sedation or anesthesia is to be administered.

Infusion—essentially, a bag of fluids to be administered intravenously; most often prepared by the Pharmacy, containing certain additives as part of the treatment plan for the patient, and may require refrigeration prior to administration; routine "fluids" may also be included in this category and are most often part of the usual stock of supplies on any given Nursing unit or department. Some fluids or Medications that come as an infusion are also photosensitive, and may require protection from light—techniques vary by hospital, but they are most often covered by a dark-colored plastic bag. Be aware of this and do not mistakenly remove and discard the bag prior to administration.

Insubordination—simply stated, it is the refusal to follow an order or directive. It may also include elements of disrespect, defiant language, and other behaviors. In many hospitals, it can be grounds for immediate termination of employment.

Isolation—the practice of placing a patient with an infectious process in a private room and requiring the use of certain equipment in order to provide care—such as gloves, mask, goggles, and/or a protective gown. The necessary precautions will be prescriptive based on how the infection is transmitted.

IV—intravenous, or what is commonly known as the "needle" (most often plastic) or "line" that goes into the patient's vein to administer fluids or Medications, or to simply provide "access". The site itself as well as any bag and tubing must be labeled and will be changed at intervals, based on your hospital's policy.

Job Description—the document that defines the responsibilities of each discipline on the team; does not usually describe technical aspects, which are most often covered by the job-specific Competency; typically used during the evaluation process to describe and quantify an employee's job performance.

Kardex—typically, a paper tool for tracking pertinent information, Orders, and events. May be a cardstock form completed by hand, or computer-generated.

Labor Unions—this is an extensive topic, but essentially, those organizations who profess to represent the rights (and, presumably the needs and wants) of their workers (Nurses, in this case), but who (in fact) can only "bargain" on wages, benefits, and working conditions. While Labor Unions certainly played a valuable role during the first half of the 20th Century in a variety of industries, there is clearly no place for them in Nursing 100 years later. Yet, as with many topics in our profession, Nurses appear all-to-willing to abdicate their power by virtually "giving up (or signing away) their rights"—thereby allowing someone else to speak for them.

Due to obvious financial gain from the annual membership dues from a large constituency of Nurses, Labor Unions will target a particular hospital and begin what is known as an "organizing campaign". They will attempt to infiltrate the entire Nursing staff by having "cards signed" as a demonstration of "support" for their desire to force a "vote". There are many rules and regulations pertaining to this process, and the impact these campaigns can have on the operations, morale, and productivity of a particular Nursing workforce is staggering, not to mention what it can do to adversely impact patient care. However, the bottom line is that invariably there are always false promises and self-serving behaviors on the part of the Union itself.

In the end, all they are able to negotiate is Wages, Benefits, and Working Conditions. That is it! Yet, the common perception among Nurses is that their power is much more far-reaching, with the potential to impact Nurse to Patient ratios, Nurse-Physician relations, decision-making (i.e. those items best addressed through a Shared Governance Model), etc. Do not fool yourselves! A Labor Union is a business, just like your hospital. They are *NOT* a charitable organization dedicated to stopping World Hunger. Ultimately, they have bills to pay, salaries to finance, and profits to be made. And, the truth is they are restricted from "bargaining" on anything more than wages, benefits, and working conditions. Period!

However, just think of the power of 1500 Nurses in a large hospital banding together (on their own) to speak up about what is best for the patient. You need to be clear—it is not necessary to pay a Labor Union as much as several hundred dollars a year in annual dues to speak for you. You have that power already. Yet, once you agree and vote "yes" to have a Union represent you, your ability to schedule an appointment with your direct supervisor (in private) to chat about issues or discuss possible improvements is gone.

Once a Union is entitled to represent you, the opportunity to have a candid conversation about what is best for Nurses and their patients has just been destroyed. From that point on, you will always have an audience of at least one—your "shop steward", who will speak on your behalf. Not to mention that a few hundred dollars of your hard-earned pay is going into *THEIR* pockets—not yours (i.e. those annual dues)! Never underestimate the power of Nursing to direct its own destiny—we already have it. What we need is Nursing Leadership. Therein we face an equal challenge!

Living Will—patients often confuse this with their "regular" Last Will and Testament, when asked the question. You may frequently find yourself explaining just what this is, so be prepared to provide accurate information. Essentially, this is their Advance Directive. (See Advance Directive)

Long Term Care—essentially, Nursing Homes and Assisted Living facilities.

LPN—Licensed Practical Nurse. LPNs are Licensed as opposed to Certified; however, in most states there are restrictions on what they can do independently. In addition, most hospitals have Policies pertaining to certain actions which cannot be performed by LPNs due the associated requirement of a "Skilled Nursing Assessment" related to that particular care, such as a Medication or Treatment. Again, know your hospital's Policies (plus the laws of your State) and understand your role in the Delegation of care for this skill level as well.

Managed Care—in simple terms, the process of "managing" healthcare to meet cost limitations and other requirements set forth by insurance companies.

Medication(s)—those medicines ordered by the Physician and which may be given on a Scheduled or As Needed (PRN) basis; they may be given orally, intravenously, rectally, topically, or through a feeding tube; may be referred to as "Meds".

Medication Error—this can be an error in the Prescribing (by the Physician), Dispensing (by the Pharmacy), or Administration (by the Nurse or designated clinician) of any Medication. Essentially, the Physician may write the wrong order (Medication, Dose, Frequency, etc), the Pharmacy may fill the order with the wrong Medication or dosage, and the Nurse/designee may give the wrong Medication to the right patient—or the right Medication to the wrong patient. There are any number of combinations of errors that can occur in this process. Your responsibility as the Nurse is to *ALWAYS* review what is commonly known as the 5 R's of Medication Administration: the *RIGHT* patient, the *RIGHT* drug, the *RIGHT* dose, the *RIGHT* route, and the *RIGHT* time.

Inherent in these steps is that you know your patient and their condition, that you have reviewed the Physician's Orders and have validated them against the Pharmacy's Medication list, *AND* that you *Pause* to review all of these elements *ONE MORE TIME* prior to administering any Medication to your patient. This must also include a review of your patient's Allergies as well. Again, if you have taken the time to review your patient's Chart, you will already be anticipating new orders. Likewise, as each Nurse performs her Chart Checks throughout the shift and every 8-24 hours (depending on your hospital's policy), such errors can be discovered before the Medication ever leaves the Medication Room.

Again, as with Falls, an Incident Report should be completed, even if the patient never actually received the Medication. Such reporting allows for trends to be discovered that can ultimately effect change and improve overall patient safety. The analysis of these events can get to the Root Cause of what may have gone wrong so that all can benefit and learn from these errors. Even when the patient did not receive the Medication, it is considered a "Near Miss" and should be reviewed.

Likewise, there are Medications that require the co-signature of another Nurse; learn what they are and follow your hospital's policy in that regard. These are typically considered high-risk Medications, with potentially lethal side effects in the event of error. And finally, another frequent issue with Medication errors is that of "Look Alike/Sound Alike" drugs, sometimes referred to as "SALADs"— meaning the names look or sound similar. There are regulations pertaining to the management of these particular Medications. Learn them as well as the process followed in your hospital to avoid such errors. If there is *NOT* a process, be the first to bring this to their attention to ensure compliance with this fundamental Standard of Care.

Mode of Urination—essentially, how you collected or observed the urine; how the patient urinated. Was it from a catheter or as a voided specimen? Was it a "Clean Catch" urine—meaning the patient used aseptic technique to clean him/herself off prior to urinating? Did you insert the catheter for a one-time collection, or did you aspirate it with a syringe from the specimen port or site of an indwelling catheter? This can be critical information, especially in the case of an infection and/or when determining the potential for a contaminated specimen. Be thorough with this aspect of Documentation.

Model, Model of Care—see Care Model.

Narcotic Count—the required accounting for, and reconciliation of, Narcotics (Opioids) and other controlled substances (Medications) that must take place on a prescribed schedule in accordance with hospital policy; typically occurs at the Change of Shift between two RNs. Always having one shift be responsible for this activity reduces the ability of *ALL* Nurses to be familiar with what is counted. Spread the wealth either by "counting" between Shifts, or by alternating this and other unit "chores" from one Shift to the other on a rotating basis, i.e. even and odd months, etc.

Narrative Note—a free-form note where the RN may record additional information that cannot be included in the prescribed fields of either paper or computerized Charting; it is imperative that any "checklist" charting match your handwritten note.

NG tube—Nasogastric Tube, used primarily for decompression and drainage of the stomach; typically inserted through the nose (and, possibly through the mouth as an orogastric tube) and requires specific techniques and precautions to ensure proper placement, up to and including an X-ray.

Hidden Bonus Pearl: when your patient vomits, do not leave their bedside, except to gather an Emesis (vomit) Basin (or bag) and a few damp washcloths. Stay at their side, wipe their face, change out the basin, and provide comfort and reassurances that they will be alright. It is completely unacceptable to walk away and "check back" on them "later". Worse yet is the Nurse who does not return at all, leaving the poor patient to manage their own cleanup—which may include a gown change, dirty linens, and/or a mess on the floor. While it may seem incomprehensible, sadly there are Nurses who fail to recognize their duty in this regard, not to mention their basic humanity and/or any degree of compassion.

Anyone who has ever been sick to their stomach, throwing up, possibly even incontinent of bowel or bladder (not able to control) due to the force of their retching should be able to appreciate how comforting it is to have a compassionate person at their side to assist, who then cleans things up once the episode has passed, when they themselves essentially fall out onto the bed—shaking, sweaty, and weak. Likewise, your patient may need Medication to control the nausea and vomiting, until the cause can be determined. This is **truly** Nursing 101! If you do not get this, you do not get it at all, and it might be best to seriously reconsider your career choice.

Normal Saline—essentially, salt water. A commonly-used fluid for intravenous administration or to irrigate a tube going into the body. There are many other formulas for IV fluids—take the time to learn what they are as well as their action in the body. Also, be sure to carefully read the labeling before "spiking" the bag to ensure you have pulled the correct one from the shelf. This is a common error when in a hurry, but inexcusable, nonetheless.

NPO—Nil Per Os—nothing to eat or drink by mouth. Remember to post a sign (See Report) at the patient's bed for this and any number of precautions—i.e. e.g. No Blood Pressure in one arm or another, Swallowing Precautions, etc. Likewise, there should be a sign posted in the bathroom if your patient is on a 24 hour urine collection and do not forget to inform all members of the Team caring for the patient so that a single voided specimen is not discarded, thus causing the entire test to be restarted. Such an error is completely unacceptable and can result in a prolonged length of stay due to a delay in discharge, pending completion of the test.

Nurse Educator—those Nurses who teach Nursing Students; may be in the clinical (patient care) setting, in the classroom, or a combination of both. One confounding factor in the Nursing Shortage is the self-imposed requirement within the world of academic Nursing that Educators must have advanced degrees. In many markets, a PhD is required. This has negatively impacted our ability to educate new Nurses; **and**, when combined with the overall Nursing Shortage, it has limited the number of available classes, thereby limiting enrollment. Yet another example of "being our own worst enemies".

Truth be told, a PhD is really not necessary to teach the basic principles of Nursing, such as how to change a bed or give a bath. Community Colleges have figured this out (in most cases), but larger Colleges and Universities with Schools of Nursing have typically set the bar just high enough to be nearly insurmountable, in terms of maintaining flow into the profession. (See Nursing Shortage)

Nursing Assistant—essentially, an extension of the Nurse. May go by a variety of titles and may or may not carry a State Certificate as a Certified Nursing Assistant; however, even with their own credentials, they are still operating under your License as a Registered Nurse, at your direction, and with your supervision via the process known as Delegation. (See Delegation)

Nursing Leadership—essentially, the hierarchy of Nurses responsible for the supervision of Bedside Nurses and all Nursing Care provided. Titles and scope of responsibility may vary from one hospital to the next. Most often, there are Nurse Managers (with or without Assistants, who may be called Assistant Nurse Managers or Patient Care Supervisors/Managers); Directors, Administrative Directors, and/or Corporate Directors (in those hospitals who have opted for a "Service Line" model, which may or may not have retained direct lines of authority to actual **Nurse** Leaders); Assistant/Associate Vice Presidents of Nursing; Chief Nursing Officers or Executives. Other titles may include Patient

Care Director, with or without an Assistant, and many other variations. (See Chain of Command, Nursing Supervisor) In a typical Service Line model, categories of care are grouped together with a "business" focus, such as all Cardiovascular, Orthopedic, Cancer Care, etc. (See Service)

Nursing Practice—the Art and Science of providing Nursing Care; may also be referred to as Clinical Practice, in generic terms. (See Art and Science)

Nursing Process—the fundamental process of Assessing, Planning, Implementing (to act or to intervene in the provision of patient care), and Evaluating Nursing Care for one or more patients. Results or Outcomes obtained should then support a modification to the Plan, if needed, or a continuation of the same Actions, as the desired goals are being met. Once all goals **have** been met, the Problem is considered resolved, and/or may also be discontinued if something else has occurred to make it no longer applicable. Included in this process is the Nursing Diagnosis following Assessment. This is not the Medical Diagnosis, but rather a determination of a real or potential deficit, or need of the patient, based upon physical/psychological/social/spiritual factors, and for which Nurses can take prescribed Actions which do not require a Physician Order.

Nursing School—the post-secondary program from which you graduate and by which you are entitled to "sit" for your State Boards; as a New Grad, you are considered to be a either a Graduate Nurse (GN) or an RN Applicant (RNA) until you have successfully passed your Boards, at which point you are licensed as a Registered Nurse (RN). Nursing Education programs vary by length and degree awarded, ranging from 2 to 4 year programs, Associate to Bachelor Degrees—in addition to many other hybrids, depending on the previous educational level of the particular candidate, such as second-degree students. (See Boards)

Nursing Shortage—the very real fact that the pool of Nurses is shrinking nationwide (for a variety of reasons), and is expected to hit a critical low within the first two to three decades of the 21st Century; this has adversely affected Nursing Education due to the decreased availability of Faculty (associated with the "greying" of the Nursing workforce in general with their associated retirement from employment), thereby creating waiting lists and/or limiting enrollment into Schools of Nursing; has resulted in the development of a variety of levels of assistive personnel to "extend" the care of the Nurse; contributes to higher Nurse to Patient ratios in some parts of the country; has resulted in the recruitment of international candidates to fill critical vacancies in certain metropolitan markets, leading to increased challenges in managing the dynamics of Cultural Diversity.

Historically, shortages have been cyclical in nature, primarily affected by economics at all levels—i.e. related to healthcare reimbursement and/or the economy in general with its impact on the available workforce. However, most agree that the shortage of the 21st Century is likely to be sustained and progressive. (See Cultural Diversity, Nurse Educator)

Nursing Supervisor—in most hospitals, the role that carries operational responsibility for the hospital during the off-shifts, in place of the Managers and Directors, and on behalf of Administration; larger hospitals may have 24/7 Supervisors on duty to manage the overall flow of patients related to Admissions and bed assignments; they work collaboratively with the Nurse Managers and report up the Chain of Command to Administration. They typically do not have responsibility for the supervision of staff, beyond the resolution of issues that may occur on a given shift.

Nursing Theorists—those Nurse Leaders who have defined a variety of philosophies related to Nursing Care for the purpose of instructing new Nurses and elevating Nursing itself to the status of a profession—something still not widely accepted just a few decades ago, at the end of the 20th Century. While valuable, these concepts rarely offer practical instruction on exactly "How to be a Nurse".

Occupied Bed—a bed with a patient in it. One comment regarding the making of beds—the sheet is *NOT* to be waved up into the air like a parachute touching down on the mattress. This stirs up dust and carries the potential to transport germs. Follow what you should have been taught in Nursing School. Lay the sheet out on one side of the bed or stretcher, and unfold it as if you were carefully opening a package.

Opioids—essentially, that class of Medications used for Pain Management, which is derived from Opium or synthetically produced as such, and historically referred to as Narcotics.

Palliative Care—the management of symptoms related to a potentially life-limiting or chronic/debilitating illness; related to reimbursement, this specialty may **still** allow the pursuit of aggressive curative treatment measures; often precedes a transition to Hospice Care when a cure is no longer possible and/or the patient/family elects to abandon those efforts.

Patent—open; may refer to a line, a tube, a drain, or some other device through which there should be flow.

Patient Handbook—a helpful resource for patients and their families that should be provided at the time of Admission and contains a wealth of information related to being a patient in that particular hospital. If your hospital no longer has one, this kind of information should at least be available on the hospital website. Also, when it comes to patient information and some key forms, these items should be available in other common languages to ensure complete understanding and to minimize liability.

Patient Representative—a person and/or department responsible for advocating for the patient as a neutral party in a variety of situations; may also be known by other names such as Patient Advocate or Patient Relations, for example. However, many hospitals have abandoned this role, and its responsibilities have now been transitioned to the Nurse Manager. This has not necessarily been a progressive move due to the potential for an absence of neutrality in resolving patient issues, as well as the typically huge workload of this position (the Nurse Manager) and the associated possibility for delays in responsiveness—not to mention the dissolution of a more consistent and centralized approach that could (or should) quickly spot trends and thereby facilitate a larger response to common issues when identified. Ideally, this position would partner with the hospital's Regulatory and Risk Management department as well as whoever is responsible for Performance Improvement (aka Quality)—which may be a separate department that goes by any of a variety of names, depending on the hospital.

Patient Satisfaction Scores—a measurement of Service Excellence by which hospitals gauge their performance within the community; typically measured on Discharged Patients via a formalized survey process using telephone solicitation or direct mail. As we move into the future of healthcare, these metrics and others have become directly proportional to reimbursement levels for hospitals, and represent a critical challenge to Nursing to produce the best possible results and outcomes, i.e. HCAHPS.

Pause—a regulatory requirement such that prior to specific care of the patient, there is a momentary pause to evaluate for the right patient, the right procedure, the right side (if applicable), etc. With Medication Administration, this would include the 5 R's (see Medication Error). This Pause or Timeout (as it is sometimes called) must be documented in the patient record, and can range from simply noting the use of two patient identifiers to the more complex details such as those before a Surgery. Know your hospital's policy, as failure to do so is not only a regulatory violation, but could also result in serious injury or death for the patient, depending on the circumstances.

Peer Review—that often (and mostly) elusive process of "peers talking to peers" in a supportive but constructive manner for the purpose of ensuring the best care of the patient, maintaining a Culture of Engagement and Clinical Excellence—or any number of reasons whereby something is not quite right or according to plan, and a course correction is needed. Yet, for whatever reason, many members of the Healthcare Team feel reluctant to view that process as a critical professional responsibility for which they are personally accountable—preferring to either ignore, gossip, run to the Manager, and/or any number of other non-productive behaviors which fail to fix the underlying issue (which in some cases potentiates the risk for patient injury or negative outcomes). This remains the greatest challenge of Leadership at all levels, and across all departments—how to facilitate a staff-driven process that is neither punitive nor personal and gets the job done before it escalates to a more serious Performance Management issue involving Disciplinary Action. (See A Word about Ethics)

Plan of Care—see Care Plan.

Policies and Procedures—essentially, the definition of how care and operations are to occur; driven by compliance and regulatory standards, as well as the Standard of Care and Evidence-Based Medicine and Nursing Practice.

Post-Anesthesia Care Unit (Recovery Room)—the area where patients are brought to recover following a surgical procedure. They are cared for until awake enough to either be taken to a second phase of recovery from where they will go home, or else to the inpatient unit for admission to the hospital where they will stay over one or more nights *OR* for potentially less than a 24 hour period, typically known as "Observation" status. This department is also known as the PACU.

Post-Op—post-operative, meaning after surgery.

Post-Traumatic Stress Syndrome (PTSD)—briefly, an intense flashback-like phenomenon in response to a highly stressful past experience that can be triggered by some event in the present that mimics or elicits those emotions as they were felt at the time of the original trauma. This can be seen with rape victims, survivors of any sort of traumatic event—natural or at the hands of another human being—as well as War Veterans who were in prison camps or in some way tortured, or simply exposed to the horrors of war.

PRBCs—Packed Red Blood Cells, or what is commonly referred to when speaking of a Blood Transfusion; ordered in terms of a "unit", as in units of blood.

Preceptor—a more experienced Nurse who orients a new Nurse to her job. Ideally, your hospital should offer a training program for this role and responsibility, as well as a defined Competency, *AND* a detailed program of goals and objectives, as well as methods and outcomes for each Preceptor and her new Orientee. The length of orientation varies by hospital and department, and should be based on previous experience; funding for such should be built into every unit's budget and should be flexible enough to guarantee that all expectations are met successfully prior to independent practice—meaning, it may be necessary to extend someone's orientation in order to ensure competency and thereby minimize potential liability. Likewise, there should be follow-up at set intervals to ensure ongoing success, as well as Engagement into the Culture of the department.

Precipitating—when pushing Medications through an IV line, the dreadful act of mixing incompatible substances such that the line clogs and is no longer usable due to the formation of particulate matter. Guarantee: you *NEVER* want to see the Doctor's face when that occurs during a Code, especially when he is the one "pushing" the Medication. If you do, you will **never** be careless in that regard again.

PRN—**Pro Re Nata**—as needed and/or as requested.

Prognosis—essentially, the expected course and/or outcome for a given disease process, based on the patient's unique clinical findings.

Progress Note—typically, the Narrative Note for the Physician, but may be multi-disciplinary (also used by the Nurse and other members of the healthcare team). Reading this should be a daily routine during your shift as it will (or should) give you a clear roadmap of the Physician's plans regarding the patient's care and prognosis.

Pulmonary Toilet—the use of Coughing and Deep Breathing to fully expand a patient's Lungs, especially after surgery or in the event of some form of pulmonary disease. May include Clapping, Cupping, or other forms of Chest Percussion. Rarely do you still see the use of Postural Drainage in the hospital setting with patients standing on their heads in the bed (a bit of an exaggeration, but that was the concept).

Pump—a variety of types and uses; when administering pain medicine, commonly known as Patient Controlled Analgesia (PCA). May also be used with feeding tubes for providing nourishment.

Reassess, Reassessment—the process of re-examining your patient from head to toe; may also be a "focused" assessment dealing with only the relevant body parts or body system, i.e. e.g. heart and/or lungs. There are (or should be) well-defined guidelines (and policies) as to the required frequency of reassessments, but they should certainly occur any time there is a real or potential change in patient condition, as well as at regular intervals throughout your shift. Negative findings (results) should be reported immediately to the Physician, with appropriate Orders given.

Regulatory Survey—the process of ensuring that a hospital or healthcare facility meets all Standards as defined by an accrediting body or organization. Again, this is a requirement for reimbursement with certain funding sources. Similar reviews occur in relation to Certification for a particular form of care within a Service Line—such as Cancer Care, Orthopedics, Bariatrics, Trauma, Stroke, Heart Attacks, etc.

Report—the age-old ritual of one shift passing on information to the next at what is commonly referred to as the "Change of Shift"; may be verbal (face-to-face) or recorded (taped). Must also occur when the patient moves from one level of care to another, such as from the Emergency Department to the ICU, or from the PACU to a Surgical ward, etc. Report should be focused, consistent, and systems-based. Ideally, it should include a review of the patient's Chart as well as the process of going room to room for each patient, and Handing Off Care from one Nurse to the next, with both the farewell of one and the introduction of the other to the patient and/or family, as well as an update and/or review of the Plan of Care (ideally with the use of a "white board"). Note: attention must be given at all times to the patient's right to privacy.

To that end, as already stated, privacy regulations (HIPAA) are complex; however, they are also clear in their intent to **not** interfere with the customary and necessary communications regarding the healthcare of the individual, especially with regard to patient safety. That said, it may be appropriate to ask the patient's permission regarding items to post on any white board and/or what to discuss when visitors are present in the room. Your hospital may facilitate this consideration by using certain key symbols on such boards that would only be understood by those involved in the care of the patient. However, even (and especially) family and friends involved in the patient's care must be instructed on those key precautions as well, to avoid inadvertent injury. This is the basis of your patient and family education and should occur throughout the course of your patient's stay in the hospital.

Finally, if you are using your "System" as you work through your shift, you will already have the basis for your Report that will be focused, clear, organized, and outcomes-driven. Again, the key to success is clarity, simplicity, and effective communication. As with most things, the more complex a process or procedure, the greater the "failure mode", and the less likely staff are to be successful. It is the responsibility of Nursing Leadership and Hospital Administration to ensure a system that enables success. Period!

RNs—Registered Nurses; the one who by law has the ultimate responsibility, in terms of Nursing Care; this includes accountability for Delegation and supervision of LPNs and Nursing Assistants or Techs; essentially, she with whom the "buck stops" (or should).

Rounds—the process of checking on all your patients; may be done at the start of a shift, known as Initial Rounds, or Hourly throughout your shift. May be a shared responsibility with an Assistant or Tech, and should be documented in patient-specific terms, not as a generic stamp that could be challenged as automated. (See Walking Rounds)

Scale—a measurement tool for evaluating (and documenting) pain (or some other patient-specific finding) that is age-specific and/or appropriate to the patient's unique ability to communicate, such as with children or the elderly, those with language or other communication barriers, the intellectually challenged, and/or those with cognitive and/or processing deficits (not able to understand or interpret higher level information). For pain assessments, this ranges from things such as a number scale to "faces" that match the number scale, in terms of the severity of the pain, i.e. a "happy face" equals a "0"or no pain, etc. The same type of scale should be used for **every** pain assessment by **every** caregiver to ensure consistency and reliability, both with the assessment itself as well as the associated and appropriate intervention based on Physician Orders. A scale is also that on which you place the patient to obtain their weight; this may be a standing scale, a "hanging" scale, or a scale built into the bed itself. (P.S. **All** patients should be weighed upon Admission, especially pediatric patients, for whom medications are most often weight-based.)

Scope of Practice—the defined range of responsibility and accountability for a given discipline; in terms of the Nurse, this is defined by the State Board of Nursing through the Nurse Practice Act. (See Board, Competency) This will also vary by area of clinical practice, in terms of skills or care that can be provided.

Service—essentially, a particular specialty in healthcare—such as Medical, Surgical, Critical Care, Orthopedic, Oncology, etc. Many hospitals have streamlined their processes around a given Service, i.e. Service Line, such that greater efficiency can be achieved related to a specific patient population, thereby improving outcomes, and concurrently (hopefully) profitability.

Service Excellence—a program directed at ensuring the best possible customer service and patient care. Includes (or should include) an element known as "Service Recovery", or the process of regaining credibility with a patient and/or family for whom something has gone wrong and/or there has been a negative outcome. This applies to simple Complaints as well as more extensive Grievances. (See Grievance)

Shared Governance—ideally, a process and a structure for effecting change directly related to Nursing Practice within a hospital or other healthcare setting. This activity should *ALWAYS* be driven by the concerns and energy of the Bedside Nurses, with oversight (but not control) by Nursing Leadership; typically comprised of a variety of committees or councils that should be structured in such a way as to allow an issue to be brought forward and then put through a process much the way a "Bill becomes a Law" in politics; these committees/councils should be comprised of Bedside Nurse members, *NOT* Nurse Leaders. A Nursing Leadership forum should be one stop in the decision-making process; however, they should *NOT* be the drivers of activity, other than what is naturally mandated via larger initiatives from organizational goals and/or regulatory or compliance directives.

These committees/councils are often grouped around many of the following categories: Clinical Practice and Standards, Education and Professional Development, Informatics, Research, Resource Management (both human capital and supplies/equipment), Retention, Ethics, Quality/Performance Improvement, and Safety. Most often, there is (or should be) a "Coordinating" body whose responsibility it is to oversee the process, and to prioritize where and how an issue enters (and proceeds through) the flow of analysis and decision-making, as well as its implementation and follow-up. Likewise, there may be specific Interdisciplinary groups and/or membership from other departments on select committees/councils (either as regular members or ad hoc) and/or there may be one group specific to Nurse-Physician relations.

These committees/councils should have by-laws related to their specific mandate that will also speak to membership and processes, in terms of voting and/or decision-making, etc. A common trap is that the same handful of Nurses is often present at and/or members of the same meetings/committees, and possibly even at or on multiple committees/councils, indicative of low enthusiasm and support by both staff and management. Ideally, this should be a robust process with widespread knowledge, understanding, participation, and outcomes. Furthermore, there may be smaller subcommittees, taskforces, etc. Overall, this process **should** tie in to the larger committee structure within the hospital such that all decision-making is focused on that one common denominator, i.e. *PATIENT CARE.*

Too often there are paralyzing redundancies on one end of the spectrum in change management, and/or inclusion failures on the other end, within the four walls of the hospital—meaning, too many folks working on the same issue at cross-purposes and/or not having the right people at the table to get the job done in the first place. Again, this ties in to the fact that healthcare is both a bureaucracy **and** a business—and neither is immune to human error and/or inefficiencies. The key to success is to assess the need, plan an ideal structure that accounts for all the nuances of a given organization, implement the model, and then continuously evaluate its success (or failure) and modify as needed. Does this sound familiar? It should! It is nothing more than the Nursing Process—one more time!

The most significant and essential sidebar consideration related to the successful implementation of a Shared Governance Model is the process by which all aspects of change are communicated. Whatever the method, there must be complete infiltration and 100% saturation down to and across all levels and all departments within the hospital or healthcare system. This means the need to have an airtight process by which no single person or entity can say, "Gee, I didn't know that!". Furthermore, there must be a comprehensive and self-sustaining mechanism for continuous feedback such that any evidence of system failure or weakness is immediately captured before any harm can come to the patient—whether the system failure is real or pre-empted.

These two aspects of project management represent real and pervasive deficits that often exist as barriers to organizational effectiveness within the hospital setting. As a Nurse, you may not be able to independently "lead the charge", but you should have both the courage and the means by which to speak up when it becomes evident that you are being "left out of the loop" in the processes that impact your ability to be successful in providing excellent patient care. Likewise, Hospital Administrators must tap into the usually immense repository of both clinical expertise and operational finesse sometimes hidden away within some (and, hopefully many) of its Nursing Leadership, and/or the Nurses themselves.

However—too often—the trend is to bring in outside consultants. This can be a catastrophic error in meeting the long-term goals of an organization. Beyond the obvious financial drain typically associated with paying for such so-called "experts", these "outsiders" are not always vested in the hospital or healthcare facility who is signing their paychecks (just like with other topics in Nursing and healthcare such as organizing activity, i.e. *Labor Unions*). Ultimately, they too are a business with the objective of making a profit. They may have helpful hints, and perhaps even an extensive database of evidence-based strategy, but in most cases the working knowledge and (most importantly) the necessary energy for effecting lasting change with positive outcomes can be found within the hospital's workforce itself. That, however, requires an engaged Executive Leadership group—brave enough to pull the strength **up** from within the broader management and leadership team, *AND*, from staff, i.e. Talent Development!

Naturally, the success of carrying on the plan of a consultant requires even greater commitment and leadership skills long after they (the consultants) leave, but all too often, the methodology of purchasing a "product" is misperceived as a total package—complete and "done" once the consultants are gone. As to be expected, over time (without leadership), the changes begin to erode and processes gravitate back to what they were before the chaos. But, all too often, key elements of what existed before have been removed and the results are now even more marginal than they were in the first place. This is a common fatal flaw in many hospitals and healthcare systems—their inability to effectively manage growth and/or change on a scale that will ensure their ultimate viability. All too often they look for the "quick fix", the "fast wins", and the "immediate gains". The cold hard truth is that Change Management is a complex Science equally mixed with Art—just like Nursing. Who better to take the reins than a Nurse! It is what we do *EVERY* day with our patients (or should)!

Staffing Plan—basically, this is the complement of staff by Discipline per shift, meaning how many Nurses, Assistants or Techs, and/or Unit Secretaries or HUCs, and /or other Disciplines are on duty, depending on the Model of Care.

Standard of Care—essentially, a universal practice or expectation related to patient care that crosses hospital and State lines. What is considered to be Best Practice and would be questioned as such in a court of law—for being followed or not, and documented as such. The absence of documentation related to meeting the Standard of Care is often what results in the winning of lawsuits when that Standard has been breached and/or accusations are made to that end—especially in the milieu of a negative and/or unexpected outcome for the patient. (See Best Practice)

STAT—Statim—Right *NOW*!!

System—a consistent way of approaching Nursing Care on any given shift, or in a particular clinical setting. Also, a particular function of the body to include all associated organs and processes, such as the Cardiovascular System. (See One Nurse's System)

Systems Format—a method for assessing and documenting a patient's condition, head to toe. Typically included are Neurologic, Cardiovascular, Respiratory, Gastrointestinal, Genitourinary, Lines, Labs, Tests, Meds, etc. or some version of the same.

Team Huddle—a recommended process for all the caregivers on a particular unit to come together for any of a variety of reasons. This may include the coordination of care following Report and Initial Rounds, for the resolution of an issue that develops during the course of a shift such as multiple admissions or a critical patient, and/or any other needs that are best resolved through communication, collaboration, and coordination of care. Depending on the kind of unit or department, other Disciplines may be involved such as Respiratory Therapy, and possibly even the Physician (such as in the Emergency Department).

Tech—similar to a Nursing Assistant, in terms of being a Nurse Extender. May vary by educational preparation, certification, and title, to include everything from a Clinical Technician with no previous healthcare background (prior to completion of a prescribed training program) to a Paramedic with extensive training and experience outside of the hospital setting.

Terminal Wean—simplistically, the process of removing life support from a patient who has been deemed as being in an unrecoverable state or having a terminal illness; will require the Advance Directive of the patient and/or the Consent of the patient, family, or next of kin, in most cases; may include the administration of pain medicines and/or other Medication for sedation to calm any degree of fear/anxiety and/or what is known as Terminal Agitation (a common phenomenon in some patients, stemming from either the disease process itself, but very often from Existential Pain). In the case of a patient on a Ventilator, this will entail the slow steady reduction in support as the Medication for sedation increases. Another complex topic for which it is best to seek support in understanding your ability to participate in such care, in terms of choosing your desired area of clinical practice.

Tongue Blade—that nasty wooden stick the Doctor uses to hold your tongue down while asking you to say "Ahh"; in the old days, ICU Nurses often used one to separate and stabilize multiple ports from a single line so they would not end up as "spaghetti"—or a tangled mess.

Toomey Syringe—a special syringe used for a variety of purposes.

Treatments—basically, care to be rendered to the patient; may be such things as Wound Care, management of tubes and drains, etc.; this is in addition to personal hygiene such as a bath and bed linen change.

Turgor—essentially, the measurement of a patient's hydration status; assessed by "pinching" up the skin (typically over the back of the hand, lower arm, or abdomen) to form a "tent", and then releasing it. Skin with "good" (or normal) turgor snaps back immediately; skin with poor turgor will remain in a tent-like position for several seconds. The latter is indicative of dehydration.

Type and Screen—a blood test that checks the patient's blood type, but does not require that units of blood be prepared or "set up" by the Blood Bank. A "Type and Cross" (meaning cross-match) must be written for blood to actually be prepared and made available for the patient. When not used, these units are "released" back into the general supply for use with another patient. Likewise, if obtained from the Blood Bank, but not initiated within a prescribed time limit, they must be returned to the Blood Bank immediately.

Similarly, once "hung" and started as a transfusion to the patient, there is also a time limit, typically no greater than 4 hours by which they must be completed. Transfusion policies and procedures are complex, and this is an area of extremely high risk. Be certain you know and understand all the requirements related to this critical element of patient care. Follow the rules and be diligent in your practice. Failure to do so could result in serious negative outcomes for your patient, up to and including death from a transfusion reaction.

Unit Secretary—the Secretary on a Nursing Unit or Department.

Vital Signs—Temperature, Pulse/Heart Rate, Respirations, Blood Pressure—and, Pain Level, as the 5th Vital Sign.

Washbasin—the standard piece of equipment used for giving your patient a bath—namely, a plastic container typically filled with water, and with which traditional soap is most often used. This may be used instead of/in conjunction with other skin care products for the purpose of cleansing (as well as protecting) the skin. There is common sense evidence that should be painfully obvious and not in desperate need of extensive research that the long-term use of a single basin without proper cleansing **between** each use could lead to the transmission of infection due to the harboring of bacteria (especially in light of so many resistant strains which no longer respond to traditional antibiotics).

Many hospitals have resorted to what is now commonly known as a "bath in a bag"—essentially a product (much like "baby wipes") that is kept (hopefully) in a warmer and used for the purpose of bathing. However, not all hospitals are willing to fund these products. If not in use in your hospital, and you must rely on the old standard of a washbasin and soap, use common sense and change them both frequently, especially when obviously old and grimy, and looking like a tub with a nasty dirty ring.

The cost of a piece of plastic and a simple bar of soap is **nothing** when compared to the high cost of a hospital-acquired infection (meaning the patient did not bring it in with them, but "caught" it while in your care). Such occurrences now impact the hospital's reimbursement for that particular patient's stay. So, in essence, Nursing is the driver of **that** bus. Get on board with your ability (and your responsibility) to effect positive outcomes for your patients through Basic Nursing Care. Another fundamental that is *NOT* Rocket Science!

Walking Rounds—the desirable process of off-going and on-coming Nurses taking a walk through their patient rooms to introduce the next shift, review the patient's Current Condition, and discuss the Plan of Care. An added benefit is that it allows for immediate attention to an urgent need with an extra pair of hands. It is a critical element in the Handoff in Care that represents Best Practice. Likewise, it can be a huge asset in facilitating accountability from one shift to the next, in terms of patient condition, stocking of supplies, and general appearances.

"When you see the natural and almost universal craving in English sick for their 'tea', you cannot but feel that nature knows what she is about. ... A little tea or coffee restores them. ... There is nothing yet discovered which is a substitute to the English patient for his cup of tea".

Florence Nightingale
Notes on Nursing, 1859

Patient Label					Date:			One Nurse's System
Room #:					Name:		Age/Gender:	
Attending:					Date of Adm:		Adm Dx:	
Resident/Intern:					Consults:		Code Status:	

HPI:	Allergies:
PMH:	Emergency Contact:

Activity	Diet	VS	I&O	BGM	Tele	O2	Isolation	Fall Risk

Surgeries	Procedures

System	Report	Changes	Time	Planned	Occurred
Neuro			08/20		
CV			09/21		
Resp			10/22		
GI			11/23		
GU			12/24		
Lines			13/01		
Labs/Tests			14/02		
Meds			15/03		
Skin/Wds			16/04		
Drns, etc.			17/05		
Family			18/06		
Misc			19/07		

Follow-up for Oncoming Shift/Plan of Care/Notes:

About the Author

Unlike traditional first-year Nursing School texts, this handbook is deliberately written in the natural voice of the Author and is intentionally conversational—if not even a lecture in itself. It is meant to be direct, slightly confrontational in terms of challenging the status quo, blatant when describing certain realities that exist in Nursing and healthcare, and ultimately a primer for all those seeking to enter the profession. Likewise, it has value for those who have fallen off the track and/or may be struggling within their own practice—simply needing the right kind of instruction that may have been missing from their initial orientation when just starting out.

As previously stated, out of convenience, the Nurse and Secretary are consistently referenced in female terms—the Physician in male terms. In no way is this meant as a sexist commentary, rather as a reflection of the traditional gender designation that was typical at the time the Author first began in her own practice in 1982. Look how far we have come! Not to mention, the ease of writing and the avoidance of he/she.

Likewise, all content solely reflects the cumulative experience of the Author over more three decades in Nursing, as validated in roles ranging from…

- o Nurse Extern on a Surgical Floor (Urology, Thoracic and Vascular) prior to graduation, to Staff Nurse on the same unit, and then to the ICU
- o to Assistant Patient Care Director of an Intermediate Care Unit, to the Post-Anesthesia Care Unit, and back to Staff Nurse to meet the demands of family
- o to Case Manager in Home Care to Clinical Manager to Regional Director, and back again to Case Manager for family
- o to Case Manager in Hospice
- o to Staff Nurse in a small rural hospital working in all departments to include Med-Surg, ICU, PACU, and the Emergency Department
- o to Patient Care Director of an Acute Pulmonary Rehabilitation Unit and a Joint Replacement/Stroke Unit
- o to Medical Center Manager of a Thoracic Cardiovascular Post-op Unit with a Thoracic Intermediate Care Unit and a Geriatric (ACE) Unit with Palliative Care and a Bariatric Unit, *AND* an Admissions Nurse for Hospice on the side
- o to Director of Clinical Operations for a start-up Hospice
- o to Staff Nurse in an Emergency Department
- o to Nurse Manager of a Freestanding Emergency Department *AND* Interim Manager of a Stroke/Medical Unit *WITH* a Behavioral Health/Detox Unit
- o to Director of Medical Nursing, with more still to come

This chronology represents human contacts too numerous to count—patients, families, coworkers, staff, Managers, Directors, Administrators, Physicians, Residents, Interns, and students from all disciplines—the sum total of a lifetime dedicated to caring for others.

For clarity and simplicity, no outside references have been used in the writing of this book, other than the quotations of Florence Nightingale appearing throughout the text at chapter end. All definitions are those of the Author, but could easily be validated with any Medical or Nursing reference. All information contained herein has been personally tested along every step in the journey of a rich and fulfilling career as a Nurse. No matter the hospital, no matter the clinical setting—these are the fundamentals that form the foundation for excellent patient care. They have been refined by the Author from one job to the next and hold true year after year, and across every hospital or healthcare system—no matter its accolades or credentials. Their intent is to finally answer the same basic question asked by so many of us in the profession—"Didn't they teach you that in Nursing 101?"—to which the response is most often an overwhelming and resounding—"*NO!*" Herein, lie the missing lessons.

As the cliché goes, "It is what it is". Neither time, nor technology can alter the essence of Nursing. It is about care, compassion, coordination, and communication—both a gift and a privilege.

The stories from each patient for whom we have cared form a rich tapestry of experience and emotion. Ideally, we learn from every case and bring that knowledge with us to the next to be applied for the benefit of all our patients and their families. Hopefully, we continue to grow and learn throughout our professional journey, moving when necessary to build on the foundation, or to add a different element to a wide range of skills and expertise. Assuming we have chosen wisely—**and** continue to feel fulfilled—we should arrive at the end of our career having become one of the **truly** Great Nurses. Again, while the choice is easy, the commitment is often a challenge—however, the rewards are unparalleled. If you are clear in your decision, and have chosen to take the plunge—**Embrace, Engage, and Enjoy!**

"I attribute my success to this—I never gave or took any excuse."

Florence Nightingale

www.ingramcontent.com/pod-product-compliance
Lightning Source LLC
Chambersburg PA
CBHW041118210326
41518CB00031B/143